Louise Stephen is a former corporate strategy consultant who was diagnosed with a life-threatening and career-ending autoimmune disease at the young age of 33. Having suffered the crippling health consequences of the condition, Louise was eventually returned to health with a kidney transplant.

Today Louise enjoys life in Melbourne with her husband and son. *Eating Ourselves Sick* is her first book.

LOUISE STEPHEN

How modern food is destroying our health

Eating Ourselves Sick

MACMILLAN
Pan Macmillan Australia

First published 2017 in Macmillan by Pan Macmillan Australia Pty Ltd
1 Market Street, Sydney, New South Wales, Australia, 2000

Cataloguing-in-Publication entry is available
from the National Library of Australia
http://catalogue.nla.gov.au

Typeset 11/18pt Sabon LT Std by Post Pre-press Group
Printed by McPherson's Printing Group
Cover concept and design by Pan Macmillan Australia

We advise that the information contained in this book does not negate personal
responsibility on the part of the reader for their own health and safety.
It is recommended that individually tailored advice is sought from your
healthcare or medical professional. The publishers and their respective employees,
agents and authors, are not liable for injuries or damage occasioned to any person
as a result of reading or following the information contained in this book.

'Vegetable Oil Consumption of the United States, 1909-1999',
The American Journal of Clinical Nutrition. Reprinted with permission.
'List of Diseases: Autoimmune and Autoimmune-Related Diseases',
www.aarda.org/autoimmune-information/list-of-diseases/. Reprinted with permission.
'Dietary carbohydrate restriction as the first approach in diabetes management: Critical
review and evidence base', *Nutrition*, 31 (2015) 1-13. Reprinted with permission.

The author and the publisher have made every effort to contact copyright
holders for material used in this book. Any person or organisation that may
have been overlooked should contact the publisher.

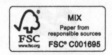

MIX
Paper from
responsible sources
FSC
www.fsc.org   FSC® C001695

*To the small hand that stopped me
from crossing the bridge*

Contents

Contents

I spent several years studying the primitive
people in various parts of the world.
And I've come as a missionary from them,
to the people of modern civilisation.
And I *beg* of you to learn of their
accumulated wisdom.
And if you do, you can have strong,
healthy bodies without so much disease
as we suffer from these days.
Weston A. Price while visiting Australia in 1936.

Foreword

The human species evolved physiologically to be hunter-gatherers, and since we performed this role around 10,000 years ago there has only been a marginal change in our physiology. The past 50–60 years have seen a marked increase in the intake of processed, packaged foods and drinks. We have been bombarded with the low-fat diet message and an explosion of pharmaceutical drugs for all manner of diseases. Despite all of this, society is getting fatter and sicker, and although our average life expectancy has peaked at around 80 there are some concerns that this will start falling because of the marked increase in 'diabesity' – the combination of diabetes and obesity. This is now close to epidemic proportions around the world, despite the bold predictions in some quarters that, in the relative future, we will be living until we are 150.

The real problem for the modern human is that we are living against our physiology, which is basically that of a hunter-gatherer. The hunter-gatherer had the acute feast of the kill, interspersed with plenty of times when food or fluid was not available, and required constant movement to obtain that food in a natural, harsh environment. The only stress experienced by the hunter-gatherer was the adrenalin rush of the kill. In our modern world, we have a constant feast with much less movement, where we are also exposed to a whole manner of synthetic chemicals and varying sources of electromagnetic radiation, not to mention complex chronic stressors. We are also living double the 'use-by date' of the hunter-gatherer, which was only around 30–40 years.

Three major groups have made billions of dollars from chronic disease or what has significantly contributed to it in the first place: the medical industry, multinational food companies and the pharmaceutical industry. But it's not just the fault of all these groups. The general public continues to practise many forms of addictive or habitual behaviour, including overeating, using legal and illegal drugs, doing sedentary jobs and following sedentary lifestyles. In addition, most people are often overwhelmed by the increasing stresses of the modern world. David Katz, the director of the Yale University Prevention Research Center once stated 'human beings living in modern society are analogous to . . . polar bears [taken] out of the Arctic and [placed] in the Sahara Desert'. He then stated, 'instead of the polar bears overheating under the Saharan sun, we are seeing human beings overeating under the Golden Arches'.

There are many books on the market telling us what is wrong with our health and giving us a variety of solutions, but Louise Stephen explains why we are where we are: historically, politically and scientifically. In *Eating Ourselves Sick*, she clearly explains the vested interests of money and power operating in many spheres of health, and how these vested interests are often part of the reason we have the extraordinary burden of chronic disease we are now seeing in our modern society. Louise asks you to challenge the collective wisdom and to question much of the accepted dogma.

Dr Ross Walker, MB BS (Hons), FRACP, FCSANZ
Consultant cardiologist
Sydney, December 2016

Introduction

In November 2002 I was 33 years old and working as a corpo-rate strategy consultant specialising in the retail and consumer markets sector. Ever since I'd sat through a sweltering summer school undergraduate strategic management class, I'd known working in this field would be right up my alley and I couldn't wait to trade the uni threads for a severe haircut and a pinstripe suit, and beat a path to the 'big end of town' where the best consulting firms had their offices. The book that had officially changed my life was *The Popcorn Report* by trend forecaster/futurist Faith Popcorn, so my grand career plan involved cutting my teeth in the consulting firms before hopefully moving into the field of trend forecasting. But, as I was to find out, the best laid plans don't always materialise. Life had other things in store. Ironically, Popcorn is famous for her core philosophy: 'If you knew everything about tomorrow, what would you do differently today?' For me the answer was 'A lot'.

Back in 2002, I loved my job in consulting although the hours, travel and high productivity under intense deadlines were likely affecting me in ways that I couldn't imagine. I was loosely aware of the idea we should eat according to the Food Pyramid – plenty of bread, pasta, rice with a few fruits and vegetables, not forgetting to eat margarine instead of butter to limit your odds of a heart attack. I rarely bothered to exercise as I was often moving around office buildings, taking stairs whenever possible or running through airports. Surrounded by the sharply dressed, image-conscious men and women that inhabit the world of consulting, I ruthlessly stayed on top of my weight. If I couldn't find the 'healthy' wholegrain bread and pastas, particularly when travelling or at client sites, I would likely find something sugary or caffeine loaded, or just not eat at all.

In terms of my health, I suffered from persistent 'brain fog' and fatigue, which I put down to a lack of either sugar, caffeine or sleep. Most of the time I had a chronic 'hacking' type of cough that X-rays and tests couldn't explain. I would recover from one chest infection, only to go down with another not long after. I would also get strange allergic-type rashes and my 'healthy' wholegrain diet would always leave me bloated and sleepy. In spite of these problems I always considered myself to be a healthy person. I was a very healthy child growing up and had never been to hospital in my life.

In my personal life, I was married and my husband and I had purchased an old home in the inner eastern suburbs of Melbourne that we had planned to renovate 'sometime down the track'. I had recently found out that I was pregnant and it seemed to us both that life was going along exactly as planned. A normal part of pregnancy testing includes a urine test, which I had dutifully turned in at the local medical clinic. I recall the doctor commenting aloud that 'the colour doesn't look too good' – apparently blood-coloured urine is not something doctors like to see. I told the doctor that my urine had taken on that hue since I'd picked up a bug a couple of months earlier. She sent it off for testing and told me to come back a few days later.

I had been working on a large project at that time and most of the project team had been infected with this bug to some degree or other. I was the sickest of all, taking two weeks off work, and had been left with yet another hacking cough, blood in my urine and, as it turned out, irreversible kidney damage. While it might seem on the surface that the bug is what caused the kidney damage, I was the only person on that project who ended up in this situation. It wasn't the bug per se but more a weakness in my own system that enabled this to happen. I had unknowingly endured the signs and symptoms of early health problems for years, and this bug was merely the straw that broke the camel's back.

When I returned to see the doctor, she referred me to a specialist who sent me for a renal ultrasound. I was about six weeks pregnant at the time and the technician was kind enough to scan my pelvis and give me a picture of my foetus. While I marvelled at the baby's tiny bean-like structure, what struck me the most was the tiny pounding heart and the realisation that I was really going to be a mum. The ultrasound was followed by a renal biopsy and diagnosis of an autoimmune disease called IgA nephropathy. Two months into my pregnancy, I was told that my kidneys would eventually fail and I would need dialysis or a transplant to stay alive.

After my diagnosis, I asked the specialist (and many specialists after that) what could have caused it. I received all kinds of casual responses, but mostly, 'It's an autoimmune disease where your body attacks itself.' Really? Bodies just go around attacking themselves for no reason? Surely there must be a little more to it. At the time, I had no choice but to accept that I was just one of the unlucky ones and that my fate was already sealed. It would be only a matter of time.

My son was born the following year and I was wisely advised by one specialist not to have any more children as it might speed up the demise of my kidneys and leave me caring for two very young children in the midst of all that kidney failure entails. I gave up the dream career I had set my sights on while still a university student because I no longer saw any point dedicating whatever time I had left with some quality of life to the pursuit of money and career goals rather than to my little boy. I renovated my house and volunteered at the kindergarten and did all the things that mums do. I hoped to at least get my son into school before I became really sick.

I spent most of 2010 in a constant state of fatigue and at the start of 2011, just as the doctor had said, my kidneys reached the end of their useful life. I decided on peritoneal dialysis via a catheter or clear tube inserted into my abdomen rather than haemodialysis via my arm, mainly because I wasn't keen on looking at blood. After the surgery to insert the catheter, I remember scarcely being able to breathe due to shock as the specialist renal nurse introduced one litre of dialysate fluid into my peritoneum for the first time. It felt very unnatural and I started to shake and cry. My husband looked on with an expression of helplessness and sadness at my new reality.

I was told by doctors that it would be easy to manage and convenient, and it would keep me going until I could find a transplant. It certainly kept me alive but it was a horrible, painful and traumatic experience. I was a terrible dialysis patient, not because I didn't want to stay alive, but because of the constant 24/7 endurance marathon of fatigue and discomfort it became. As a mother to a young child and with little support, it became harder and harder to juggle all of life's responsibilities while sinking into quicksand at the same time.

Nobody tells you about the constant lethargy, the loss of appetite, the jumpy legs, the skin sores, the body odour, the forgetfulness, the nausea, the inability to sleep, the loss of interest in everything. Nobody tells you about the erratic blood chemistry and how impossible it can prove to keep it within reasonably safe parameters. In May, 2012 I was privileged to receive a matching kidney from a deceased donor and it came not a moment too soon. By the time I had my transplant I had become drawn and spent most of my time resting or sleeping. I really didn't know how much longer I would last, and it was a far cry from my life as a corporate consultant jetting all over the place. I remember the feeling I had as I was being wheeled into the theatre for my transplant. It was the feeling of just not caring about what might happen to me anymore. Death on the operating table might offer some relief from my horrible reality.

Fortunately, my transplant went well and I was discharged from hospital within the week. I can still remember blinking into the sunshine as I exited the hospital, holding my stomach like a precious cargo as I tentatively shuffled toward the patient pick-up. Sitting on a street bench, I struggled to process the chain of events that had just transpired. Somewhere a selfless family was grieving the unexpected loss of a loved one, while I had just received a second chance at life. After months of recovery and a couple of setbacks, I was able to take a beach holiday. On dialysis I was unable to go swimming on hot days (despite the convenience of living opposite the beach) or take holidays, so to be able to soak in the clear waters off Whitehaven Beach in the Whitsunday Islands was like being reborn.

Looking at me now, one would hardly believe I had been so sick. I must take anti-rejection medications every day but I look and feel totally normal and healthy. Several years have passed, but not a day goes by where I don't think of my donor and feel gratitude for the priceless gift they gave me. Today I consider myself to be among the many, mostly female 'corporate refugees' who have succumbed to some type of chronic disease (such as autoimmunity) leaving their careers, earning ability and human potential in tatters. Do I live my life differently to before? Of course.

Home cooking with fresh, healthy ingredients is non-negotiable. Soft drinks and processed junk foods are not included in my shopping trolley. Seed oils and gluten are also out – for reasons you will read about in this book. I recognise stress for what it is and manage it accordingly and exercise is for enjoyment. Life is simply too short to be doing activities you dislike. Sleep also ranks highly on my list of essentials.

Autoimmune disease related organ failure is not the human experience that I wanted or expected. And it's not the human experience that I would wish upon any other person. But unfortunately, chronic disease such as heart disease, cancer, metabolic syndrome and auto-immunity, and the pain and suffering they visit upon us, will be the experience of many adults and increasing numbers of children as time goes on – unless people start to become educated about the importance of health, take responsibility for their own health and that of their children, and understand what causes chronic disease and how it can be prevented, partially or substantially ameliorated, and in some cases reversed. This is not altogether easy, as many different organisations and individuals in our society would like to tell us how to run our health. Many of them have agendas of their own, both seen and unseen. So whom do we trust? In my case, I had to learn to trust myself, my own reading and analysis, and my own instincts.

My experience of being told that autoimmune disease 'just happens' to some people left me feeling confused and helpless. How could my body just attack itself? Knowing how hyper-intelligent the human body is and the extraordinary lengths it will go to in order to survive, this casual explanation just didn't add up. I remember one doctor telling me my condition was genetic, that I was born this way.

Other unhelpful offerings from strangers included I was prob-ably being punished by God for something I'd done wrong; that I needed to merely 'think' myself well again; that I'd done some-thing bad in another life and was being punished in this one; and that because kidney beans are red and shaped like kidneys, I just needed to eat large amounts of them and I would be cured.

None of these scenarios made any logical sense to me, and the mystery of why my life was going to be cut short, remained just that, a mystery. It wasn't until I watched a documentary on a remote hill tribe from New Guinea that had mostly refused contact with outside individuals that I started to see things in a new light.

The featured tribe had decided to allow a group of medical anthropologists to study them. This tribe had never consumed foods outside of the area in which they lived. The medicine man was responsible for the health and wellbeing of tribe members. They had never used pharmaceuticals. They shunned contact with outsiders and they were located in a very remote and rugged location, far away from the trade routes. Among other findings, the researchers discovered that there was no apparent history in the group of chronic diseases such as those at epidemic levels in the West. They mostly worried about infections, animal attack, violent tribal disputes or serious physical injuries. The medicine man appeared puzzled by the mere concept of chronic disease.

I realised at that point that autoimmune disease, or for that matter any chronic disease, most likely did not 'just happen' to people. Our environment has been playing a major role in the explosive growth of chronic disease all along.

I was further intrigued when I read the classic *Nutrition and Physical Degeneration* by Weston A. Price (1870–1948), an American dentist who surveyed the physical differences between isolated and modernised indigenous peoples in the 1930s. Price found that isolated groups enjoyed excellent physical and mental health, were largely resistant to illness, were physically robust, and their teeth straight and free of decay. If one of these people consumed the refined wheat, sugar and seed oil products made available due to trade, the negative impact on their health was quite profound.

Some among the subsequent generations were born with birth defects, were extremely susceptible to infections and developed behavioural problems that the indigenous people had never seen before. Some also suffered from inflammatory conditions such as arthritis and had malformed physical features, including the face and dental arch, as well as rotted and gap-filled teeth. The women suffered from fertility problems and started to have trouble giving birth due to narrowed birth canals, indicating that bone structure beyond the face was being affected. Price deduced that sugar and refined wheat had robbed these people of their immunity, making them more susceptible to contracting infectious diseases such as tuberculosis. The loss of immunity to dental caries and inability to obtain dental care led some of these people to take their lives rather than suffer the pain of abscessed teeth. Tragically, these indigenous populations were painfully aware that the 'white man's food' delivered to them via the trade winds was responsible for the shocking decline in their health and communities, and they raised their observations and concerns with Price throughout his travels.

While the scientific insight was not as advanced as it is today, and availability and sophistication of formal diagnostic testing was limited, Dr Price could not help but notice the striking similarities in terms of disease susceptibility across all populations studied, which appeared to be in direct alignment with the introduction of specific store foods.

Almost 80 years later, the worst fears of many of Price's research subjects have been well and truly realised. According to the World Health Organization, up to 40 per cent of Pacific Islanders have been diagnosed with cardiovascular disease, diabetes or hypertension (high blood pressure), which account for three-quarters of all deaths across the region. American Samoa boasts an obesity rate of 80 per cent (among women) and an adult diabetes rate of 47 per cent. Iron, iodine and vitamin A deficiencies are rife. Indigenous Australians are three times more likely than non-indigenous to have type 2 diabetes and 38 times more likely to require a lower limb amputation as a result. Cancer and type 2 diabetes rates have dramatically increased among the Inuit population. The tragic statistics go on and on with no end in sight.

Might Weston Price's study subjects turn out to be the canary in the coalmine? Were they unwitting early victims in some type of food-based human extinction event that will eventually swallow us all? Could it be that in spite of their incredible ability to survive a high-risk hunter-gatherer existence for in some cases tens of thousands of years, they are unable to survive the impact of a diet based on sugar, refined wheat and seed oil?

Is there any hope for them?

I will never know the exact cause of my own disease. What I do know is this: contracting a life-threatening disease motivated me to understand more about my own health and my curiosity about the sorts of things that lead to improved health. Over and over, it came back to the food we put in our bodies. Looking closely at the parlous state of our modern-diet led to me wonder: is there any hope for us?

The Wayback Machine

You may have heard of the Wayback Machine, the digital archive of the internet that captures and stores digital content over time. It's a useful tool for catching out slippery politicians or raking over someone's digital past. Named for the WABAC time machine featured in *The Rocky and Bullwinkle Show*, the overarching goal of the Wayback Machine is to eventually archive the entire internet.

The interesting thing about the Wayback Machine is that in generations to come people will be able to revisit media content of our time and analyse our thoughts and opinions. They will be able to read about the obesity crisis, the explosion of autoimmunity, the increase in the incidence of cancer. They will read about the introduction of foods containing genetically modified organisms (GMOs) and how, not unlike the millions of tonnes of herbicides and pesticides that were sprayed on the global food supply, they were considered safe as defined by industry 'until proven otherwise'. They might be appalled at how naïve and foolish their ancestors were and wonder how we could have stood en masse and in silence, waiting patiently for the 'science to ripen'. They might wonder why we did little more than twiddle our thumbs while allowing so many things to get so out of control so quickly. One thing is for sure, they won't forgive us – and nor should they.

Weston Price showed us that standing by and letting things get out of control is nothing new. In what might be described as a rudimentary version of the Wayback Machine, Price provided us with the photographic and documentary evidence of indigenous populations who were in existence at around the same time the 'blessings of civilisation' began to take hold in their environments. Thus he was able to capture many images of people who had never partaken of such 'blessings' and who boasted extraordinary health, along with those who had indulged, and consequently succumbed to physical and mental degeneration.

Price's documentary evidence clearly shows that his subjects were painfully aware of the effect modernisation was having on their health and wellbeing, and on their family units and communities in general. Indeed, Price noted with regard to a group of Indigenous Australians: 'One can scarcely visualize . . . the distress of a group of primitive people . . . compelled to live in a very restricted area, forced to live on food provided by the government, while they are conscious that if they could return to their normal habits of life they would regain their health and again enjoy life.'

No matter where he travelled in his pursuit of knowledge and understanding, Price observed the impressive overall health and disease resistance (to local pathogens) of the indigenous peoples committed to traditional eating habits, and the failing health and limited disease resistance of those that either by necessity or desire switched to modern foods. This was the case among groups in Africa, northern Scotland, the Pacific Islands, Australia, the United States and New Zealand.

THE WORDS OF WESTON A. PRICE

Here is a selection of Price's findings among the numerous groups he visited and examined, couched in the language of his own time. Of the African people, he wrote:

> In one of the most efficiently organized mission schools that we found in Africa, the principal asked me to help them solve a serious problem. He said there was no single question asked them so often by the native boys in their school as why it is that those families that have grown up in the mission or government schools were physically not so strong as those families who had never been in contact with the mission or government schools . . .

> Dr. Anderson who is in charge of a splendid government hospital in Kenya, assured me that in several years of service among the primitive people of that district he had observed that they did not suffer from appendicitis, gall bladder trouble, cystitis and duodenal ulcer. Malignancy was also very rare among the primitives . . .

> An examination of 320 teeth of ten individuals revealed twenty teeth with caries, or 6.3 per cent. It is significant that all of the carious teeth were in the mouth of one individual, the cook. The others all boarded themselves and lived on native diets. The cook used European foods.

Of the Gaelic people in northern Scotland:

> The elderly people were bemoaning the fact that the generation that was growing up had not the health of former generations. I asked what their explanation was and they pointed to two stone grinding mills which they said had ground the oats for oatcake and porridge for their families and preceding families for hundreds of years . . . They told us with great concern of the recent rapid decline in health of the young people of this district . . .
>
> My examination of the children in this community [the Isle of Skye] disclosed two groups, one living exclusively on modern foods, and the other on primitive foods. Those living on primitive foods had only 0.7 carious teeth per hundred, while those in the group living on modern foods had 16.3 or twenty-three times as many.

Of the South Sea Islanders:

> The Tahitians are . . . fully conscious . . . of their rapid decline in numbers and health.
>
> Many of the island groups recognize that their races are doomed since they are melting away with degenerative diseases, chiefly tuberculosis. Their one overwhelming desire is that their race shall not die out. They know something serious has happened since they have been touched by civilization.

Of the Torres Strait Islanders:

> In their native state they have exceedingly little disease. Dr. J. R. Nimmo, the government physician in charge of the supervision of this group, told me in his thirteen years with them he had not seen a single case of malignancy [cancer] . . . among the entire four thousand native population. He stated that during

this same period he had operated on several dozen malignancies for the white population, which numbers about three hundred. He reported that among the primitive stock other affections requiring surgical interference were rare.

Of the Australian Aborigines:

This group . . . are dependent almost entirely on the food provided by the mission and the government. The official in charge had spent fifty years in devoted service to these native people. We found him exceedingly sad because of the very rapid breakdown that was in progress among the natives in his care . . . We were advised that deaths occurred very frequently from tuberculosis. This reservation does not provide the natives with natural hunting grounds capable of providing the people with animal life for food . . .

The cook on the government boat was an aboriginal Australian from Northern Australia. He had been trained on a military craft as a dietitian. Nearly all his teeth were lost. It is of interest that while the native Aborigines had relatively perfect teeth, this man who was a trained dietitian for the whites had lost nearly all his teeth from tooth decay and pyorrhoea . . .

On Murray Island . . . the natives were conscious of a danger from the presence on the island of a store providing imported foods. This had been so serious a problem that there was a question whether it would be safe for us to land, since on the last visit of the government officials, blood was almost shed because of the opposition of the natives to the government's program.

In reference to a Dr Josef Romig, a surgeon with 36 years' experience among traditional and modernised Inuit and Native Americans, he wrote:

He stated that in his thirty-six years of contact with these people he had never seen a case of malignant disease among the truly primitive Eskimos and Indians, although it frequently occurs when they become modernized . . .

He found similarly that the acute surgical problems requiring operation on internal organs such as the gall bladder, kidney, stomach, and appendix do not tend to occur among the primitive, but are very common problems among the modernized Eskimos and Indians. Growing out of his experience, in which he had seen large numbers of the modernized Eskimos and Indians attacked with tuberculosis, which tended to be progressive and . . . fatal as long as the patients stayed under modernized living conditions, he now sends them back when possible to primitive conditions and to a primitive diet, under which the death rate is very much lower than under modernized conditions. Indeed, he reported that a great majority of the afflicted recover under the primitive type of living and nutrition.

Of the New Zealand Maori:

The breakdown of these people comes from when they depart from their native foods to the foods of modern civilization, foods consisting largely of white flour, sweetened goods, syrup and canned goods. The effect is similar to that experienced by other races after using foods of modern civilization.

Price reminds his readers that while we might seek to mock the government officials who provided the indigenous populations with the modernised foods that consequently destroyed their health, we should remember that Western officials and bureaucrats were themselves under a similar yoke. They just didn't know it.

Price's findings on foods

At this point it's worth examining a summary of the traditional foods consumed by each of the groups together with the modernised foods made available to other local groups, and the health conditions the indigenous people suffered as a result. There is a notable disparity between the indigenous diets pursued by each group, some following a Paleo or hunter-gatherer style of eating, others a diet high in dairy or animal fats. In addition, indigenous diets did not include processed foods. Not one of the groups was remotely following the standardised carbohydrate-heavy 'food pyramid' commonly recommended in Western countries at the time; on the contrary, their diets were rich in protein, fats and unprocessed plant foods.

Group	Traditional foods	Introduced foods	Introduced health conditions
Swiss from Lötschental Valley – 1931	Nutrient-dense hand-threshed, stone-ground whole-rye bread; nutrient-dense grass-fed cow's and goat's milk, cheese and butter; soups, stews, small amounts of meat and vegetables during warmer months	White flour, sugar, jams, marmalades, jellies, syrup, canned goods, chocolate	Substantial dental caries, extreme susceptibility to tuberculosis, low immunity, deformed dental arches
Gaels from the Isle of Lewis – 1931–32	Lobsters, crabs, oysters, clams, fish, fish organs, eggs, marine plants, oats (locally grown in highly fertilised soil) in the form of oatcakes and porridge	White bread and flour, sugar, jams, marmalades, syrup, canned goods, chocolate, coffee, canned vegetables	Rampant tooth decay, extreme susceptibility to tuberculosis, low immunity, deformed dental arches

North American Indians – 1933	Fish, fish eggs, seaweed, organ and tissue meats from wild animals such as moose and deer, dried berries, ground nuts, dried tree buds	White flour, commercial vegetable fats, jams, marmalade, syrup, sweetened goods, confections, pastries, and canned vegetables	Rampant tooth decay, crowded teeth, deformed dental arches, narrow nostrils and mouth breathing, susceptibility to tuberculosis, childhood and adult arthritis, deformities, extreme population reduction, impaired reproductive capacity, prenatal injury and increased need for surgical intervention during childbirth, malignancies, increased susceptibility to general infections
Inuit people – 1933	Fish, fish eggs, seal oil, whale organs and skin, kelp, caribou, berries, flower blossoms, liberal use of fresh organ meats	As above	As above
South Sea Islanders – 1934	Fish, seafood, crab, coconut, shellfish, octopus, land-grown plants, limited amounts of taro, seeds and breadfruit	White flour, sugar, sugar products, sweetened goods, canned foods, polished rice	Rampant tooth decay, abscessed teeth, gingival infections, deformed dental arches, extreme population reduction, susceptibility to tuberculosis, measles, smallpox, depressed reproductive capacity

African cattle tribes – 1935	Freshwater fish and animals, cow's milk, blood, meat, organs, insects, plants, vegetables, fruits, elephant meat, bananas, salt (a prized mineral)	Sugar, white flour, canned goods, polished rice	Tooth decay, facial deformities and narrowing of the face and dental arches, nutritional deficiency disorders, greatly reduced reproductive efficiency, extreme population reduction, loss of disease resistance and extreme susceptibility to 'Western' disease processes
Indigenous Australians – 1936	Fish, shellfish, dugong, kangaroo, wallaby, grubs, insects, roots, stems, leaves, seeds, berries, seaweed, kelp, small rodents, birds and birds' eggs	Sugar, white flour, canned foods	Depressed reproductive capacity, facial deformities, extreme disease susceptibility, inability to breastfeed infants, physical deformities, tuberculosis, deformed dental arches, abscessed and rotted teeth
New Zealand Maori – 1936	Sea animals, marine plants, marine and land birds and eggs, seeds, plants, vegetables, grubs, fern roots, kelp	White flour, sugar, canned foods, sweetened goods, syrup	Prenatal injury, undersized and deformed children, physical deformities, tuberculosis, tooth decay, deformed dental arches, rapid decline in reproductive capacity

The common theme that underpins the dramatic about-face in the health of every one of Price's indigenous groups is the shift from the traditional diet to one derived from the raw materials of sugar, white flour, vegetable fats (hereinafter referred to as seed oils), polished rice and processed canned foods. Price notes that the administrators of the trading vessels that brought these foods to the Pacific Islands *were instructed* to give Western food in exchange for island goods, such as copra, 90 per cent as sugar and white flour, and only 10 per cent in clothing or other products.

A return to health

Price makes numerous references to the fact that many indigenous men, women and children reclaimed their previous good health when they returned to their traditional diets and no longer consumed processed foods. In other words, the decline in health and immunity, and the onset of disease, was in many cases partially or fully reversible.

This assertion was tested under controlled conditions many years later by Australian nutrition researcher Kerin O'Dea. In 1982, O'Dea returned a group of overweight and pre-diabetic or diabetic Indigenous Australians to their ancestral homelands to partake in their traditional hunter-gatherer diet of mostly kangaroo, inland fish and yams. Not surprisingly, the blood-glucose profile of the study participants improved, and some were able to reverse their type 2 diabetes.

The observation that sickness, disease and poor health could ensue simply through the replacement of a traditional diet with one that included high amounts of sugar and refined wheat was not limited to the detective skills of Weston Price. Researchers have witnessed the same phenomenon in other locations around the world. In 2015, the tiny Pacific Island territory of Tokelau was named as having the world's highest prevalence of type 2 diabetes among adults. Before the establishment of trading posts on the island in the mid-1970s, the traditional diet of the Tokelauan people had consisted of fish, coconuts and breadfruit. Health problems were limited to skin diseases and infectious diseases. The arrival of imported foods resulted in a sevenfold increase in sugar consumption and a roughly sixfold increase in flour consumption, not to mention weight gain, cancer, diabetes, hypertension, heart disease and gout.

In another well-known study of the isolated Kitavan people, who live in the Trobriand Islands near Papua New Guinea, researchers noted a distinct lack of cardiovascular disease, stroke, hypertension and diabetes. Dementia and memory loss among tribal elders (one as old as 96) were also notably absent. Obesity and being overweight were also non-existent, and researchers were unable to find a single case of acne, even among the high-risk group of those aged between fifteen and 25. Kitavans are subsistence horticulturalists whose traditional diet (while high in carbohydrates) consisted of fish and seafood, root vegetables, fruit, vegetables and coconuts. Access to 'store foods' such as sugar, cereals, fats, alcohol and dairy was negligible, and accounted for less than 0.2 per cent of food intake compared with 75 per cent in a European country such as Sweden.

The Tsimané people of the Bolivian Amazon still live a lifestyle that is a cross between horticulturalist and hunter-gatherer, subsisting on corn, rice and cassava together with wildlife sourced from the jungle. They rarely participate in the cash economy and have limited access to store foods such as refined sugar, wheat and seed oils (although they do access fruit and some sugar cane).

Vaccinations arrived in the 1990s but parasites and bacterial infections are still a problem, and life expectancy is short, at about 50 years. There are, however, no recorded cases of cardiovascular disease, cancer (breast, prostate, ovarian, colon, testicular) or asthma. Autoimmune disease is breathtakingly rare: health workers found (out of a population of 12,000) one case of rheumatoid arthritis (0.008 per cent), one case of lupus (0.008 per cent) and eleven cases of vitiligo (0.09 per cent). Hypertension, at epidemic levels in the West, is also exceedingly rare. While the blessings of Western 'civilisation' are absent from the Tsimané community, so too is the scourge of chronic disease.

Compare these statistics to Australia with an estimated 428,000 or around 2 per cent of the population (mostly women) affected by rheumatoid arthritis at a cost of $273.6 million for the medications alone. Lupus is believed to affect over 20,000 Australians and New Zealanders (nine out of ten patients are women). Rates among indigenous Australians are understood to be much higher. Vitiligo is understood to affect 1 to 2 per cent of the global population.

Numerous lines of inquiry clearly demonstrate that the decline in health and fertility of indigenous people around the world is intimately connected to the introduction of the ubiquitous store foods – sugar, refined wheat and seed oils.

The modern movement

Almost 80 years after Weston Price recorded his observations, many 'Westerners' who have actively removed sugar, flour, seed oils and processed foods from their diets, and replaced them with nutrient-dense 'real foods', are claiming either partial or full remission from a range of chronic health symptoms and conditions, including metabolic syndrome symptoms and type 2 diabetes. This phenomenon, however, is often dismissed and even ridiculed by various 'traditional' health authorities that allege to be in the business of protecting our health. But if the ability of specific foods to interfere with our health has been known for so long, why were those foods allowed to eventually dominate our food supply? Where does the responsibility for such a decision lie?

The Wayback Machine circa 2060 will reveal one of two possibilities. The people, tired of waiting for the miracle cures promised by science and charlatans alike, opened their eyes to the possibility that health was always about prevention and the real key had been sitting under their noses all along. And they decided to make a change.

Or they didn't.

2

How did *we* get so fat and sick?

According to the World Health Organization, chronic diseases (also known as non-communicable diseases) are illnesses of long duration and usually slow progression. The four leading chronic diseases are cardiovascular diseases that lead to heart attack and stroke, cancer, diabetes, and chronic respiratory diseases such as asthma. The World Economic Forum predicts that by 2030, a mere thirteen years from now, chronic disease could kill 52 million people per year and cost the global economy US$47 trillion. It has the potential to bankrupt health systems and slow global economic growth. People are getting sicker younger, and of great concern is the way families, communities, countries and economies are losing their most productive people to these debilitating illnesses.

Add to the diagnosed cases the sheer number of people who just feel unwell all the time and – despite following advice issued by doctors, diet experts and various organ- or disease-based organi-sations – never seem to feel or get any better. Consider as well the increasing numbers of children and young people with chronic diseases, allergies, eczema, intolerances, obesity, depression, infer-tility and other symptoms of physical breakdown. The financial cost of this crisis pales in the face of individual suffering and the sheer loss of human potential.

We are constantly told by 'traditional' health authorities to eat more grains, choose low-fat and no-fat food and cut down on 'treats'. The inconvenient truth, however, is that in an era where we have more scientists, doctors, medical personnel, dietitians, nutri-tionists, hospitals, pharmaceuticals, community support services, health bureaucrats, medical researchers and facilities, and more government investment in health, we have never collectively been fatter or more chronically diseased in the known history of the human race. According to the World Economic Forum, the United Kingdom's National Health Service is the world's fifth largest employer, boasting 1.7 million employees, not far behind the People's Liberation Army of China with 2.3 million staff, and still the British people continue to get fatter and sicker.

And the problem is set to get much worse.

Cancer

In early 2014, the World Health Organization announced that cancer cases are expected to increase by 57 per cent globally within the next two decades, with an economic cost of US$1.16 trillion. Cancer has now overtaken cardiovascular disease as the number one cause of death of men in the United Kingdom, Belgium,

Denmark, France, Israel, Luxembourg, the Netherlands, Portugal, Spain, Slovenia and San Marino, and researchers project that a tipping point, where cancer deaths will outnumber deaths from cardiovascular disease, is rapidly approaching. Billions of dollars have been spent on Richard Nixon's 'war on cancer', launched in 1971, but maybe it's time to conclude that cancer has won not just many of the battles but the entire war.

Dr Christopher Wild, director of the World Health Organization's International Agency for Research on Cancer (IARC) perhaps sums up the situation best: 'Despite exciting advances ... we cannot treat our way out of the cancer problem ... More commitment to prevention and early detection is desperately needed to ... address the alarming rise in the cancer burden globally.' According to cancer specialists, obesity is now set to overtake smoking as a key cause of cancer in the West. The links between obesity and cancer are now clear: obesity increases the risk of ten of the most common cancers in women including post-menopausal breast cancer and, cancer of the rectum, colon, liver, gall bladder, pancreas, endometrium, ovary, kidney and thyroid.

One of the most interesting features of untouched indigenous groups studied by researchers over the years is the virtual absence of cancer – a health issue that appears in alarming numbers in Western populations. Indeed, one in two British people born after 1960 can now expect to have cancer in their lifetime. While we are often led to believe that cancer is still a great mystery probably rooted in genetics, research from more recent times lines up the major contributors to the main cancers that plague us. This research might help explain the gulf between the lack of cancer in Dr Price's research subjects and the 'half the population' figures we can expect today.

Decades of cancer research was aggregated and analysed by Professor Max Parkin and published in 2010. It shows that we are surrounded by lifestyle and environmental factors that contribute to the 100 diseases we call cancer: tobacco; obesity, driven by processed 'displacing' foods; lack of the nutrient density typically drawn from 'real food'; alcohol consumption; chemicals used in workplaces; sunbeds; viral and bacterial infections such as human papilloma virus, Epstein Barr virus, cytomegalovirus and *Helicobacter pylori*; red and processed meat; radiation; a low-fibre diet; inactivity; not breastfeeding; salt; and hormone replacement therapy. Most, if not all of these factors were unknown to the untouched indigenous groups, particularly cigarettes, alcohol, chemicals, obesity-inducing foods and foreign infections. Further research released in 2015 showed that such environmental factors may account for up to 70–90 per cent of the cancers we experience.

WHAT IS METABOLIC SYNDROME?

Metabolic syndrome, also called 'the' metabolic syndrome or syndrome X, is a cluster of conditions – excess abdominal weight, high blood triglycerides (fats), low levels of HDL ('good') cholesterol, hypertension (high blood pressure), high blood glucose and insulin resistance. Together, they increase the risk of developing type 2 diabetes and/or cardiovascular disease – possibly leading to heart attack or stroke.

Some people are genetically predisposed to developing metabolic syndrome, but it's also considered a lifestyle disease, linked to overeating (or, as we will see, eating the wrong things), poor sleep and lack of exercise.

Type 2 diabetes

Diseases for which metabolic syndrome is the precursor, such as type 2 diabetes, are also exploding around the world. In Australia, 1 million people have been diagnosed with the condition. China, one of the world's leading sugar importers and the world's largest consumer of omega-6 soybean oil, has earned the title of 'world capital' of type 2 diabetes, where cases have tripled in just one decade and now affect more than 90 million people. Chinese consumption of seed oils has increased by 2000 per cent since 1990, and today one-third of Chinese adults are overweight compared to an insignificant proportion 25 years ago. Sadly, type 2 diabetes today touches more young people in China than in the United States, and this has been put down to carbonated soft drinks and snacking. Diabetes costs China around US$28 billion per year, and this is expected to rise as more cases are detected.

WHAT IS INSULIN RESISTANCE?

After we eat, the glucose levels in our blood rise. In response, the pancreas releases the hormone insulin into the blood, which in normal circumstances stimulates cells throughout the body to take up the glucose and return levels in the blood to normal.

In insulin resistance, although the pancreas produces insulin as normal, the cells don't respond and blood glucose stays high. This feeds back to the pancreas, which increases production of insulin, leading to high blood levels of insulin (hyperinsulinemia) as well as of glucose.

WHAT IS TYPE 2 DIABETES?

When insulin resistance persists over a number of years and the pancreas continues to overproduce insulin in an effort to bring down blood-glucose levels, the pancreatic cells eventually wear out and can no longer produce any insulin at all. About 50 per cent of the pancreatic cells will be ineffective by the time a diagnosis of type 2 diabetes is made. This means that a combination of useless insulin and not enough insulin allows blood glucose to rise and stay high.

When this high sugar blood is bathing every organ, damage is inevitable. Late-stage complications of type 2 diabetes include heart attack and stroke, retinal damage and possible loss of vision, kidney damage and amputations.

Type 2 diabetes is a lifestyle disease but there is a strong genetic component. This means that two people might have the same poor diet and inactive lifestyle but only the one with the genetic predisposition develops type 2 diabetes. The standard initial medical advice is to improve the diet and increase exercise, but most people under a doctor's care eventually end up taking some form of medication.

India comes second to China with more than 61 million diabetics, a number expected to increase to 100 million within fifteen years. More rural people (34 million) than urban people (28 million) are affected with type 2 diabetes. This is because rural Indians consume very high levels of high-carbohydrate cereal grains, and at least half of one group studied by researchers consumed no green leafy vegetables, fruits, nuts or meats. The excessive carbo-hydrate diets of the rural Indians may be just as problematic as the increasingly Westernised urban diet. India is also the world's fourth-largest consumer of omega-6 soybean oil after Brazil and the United States. Soybean oil consumption, which has exploded in China, India and the United States, has been shown in mouse studies to be a greater cause of obesity and diabetes than fructose (see page 126).

Alzheimer's disease

Alzheimer's disease is the most common form of dementia. The brains of people with Alzheimer's exhibit two particular abnormalities: amyloid plaques and neurofibrillary tangles. Plaques are deposits of amyloid beta peptides (small proteins – strings of around 40 amino acids) outside the cells in the grey matter. These occur in small numbers as a normal brain ages, but in Alzheimer's they are numerous. Neurofibrillary tangles are clumps of tau protein inside brain cells that may interfere with their normal functioning.

'Type 3 diabetes' is a term increasingly used for Alzheimer's, to indicate that it can in some ways be considered a metabolic disease. It was coined in response to research findings from Brown Medical School in the United States, which recognised that the brain, not just the pancreas, could produce insulin. Both insulin resistance and insulin-like growth factor (IGF-1) have been identified as playing a key role in the progression of Alzheimer's disease. In addition, researchers have discovered that many people with type 2 diabetes have amyloid deposits in their pancreas that are similar to the amyloid plaques found in the brain tissue of Alzheimer's sufferers. In 2015 American researchers at Washington University found that elevated blood glucose could rapidly increase amyloid beta levels in the brain, while a 2013 study at Tulane University in Louisiana found that high blood glucose could make amyloid beta protein more toxic to brain cells. More than 400 trials for Alzheimer's medications took place between 2002 and 2012, resulting in a failure rate of 99.6 per cent – among the highest for a disease. Only one drug, memantine, has been approved since 2004.

Given the role of insulin resistance in Alzheimer's and dementia-type conditions it would seem that diet over one's lifespan would appear to be a bigger risk factor than simply age. In 2015, the Office of Health Economics, in research carried out on behalf of Alzheimer's Research UK, estimated that 32 per cent of babies born in the United Kingdom during 2015 would develop dementia within their lifetime. The outlook for females was significantly worse, with 37 per cent likely to develop the condition over 27 per cent of males. If such projections prove accurate, the combined health burden of type 2 and type 3 diabetes on the British taxpayers and health system will prove insurmountable in the coming years.

WHAT IS AN AUTOIMMUNE DISEASE?

In an autoimmune disease, the body mistakes its own cells for invaders and attacks itself.

In the normal immune system, white blood cells called T cells have surface receptors that allow them to recognise the difference between antigens (any molecule that can bind to a receptor and cause an immune response) from our own cells (called self-antigens) and those from foreign invaders. When they encounter an invader, they instruct other white blood cells, called B cells, to produce antibodies that attack and neutralise the invader. B cells also produce

---

cytokines, which are signalling molecules that cause an inflammatory response designed to allow the body to fight infection.

Vaccines work on the principle of introducing an antigen (which could be as little as a single protein) without any infectious capacity into the blood. In response, the body produces antibodies that, in the event of an infectious agent entering the body, recognise that specific invader and prevent infection.

In autoimmunity, T and B cells mistakenly recognise self-antigens as foreign and produce antibodies against them. These antibodies then attack a certain part of the body, causing inflammation and damaging tissues. Which part of the body they attack (and thus which autoimmune disease they produce) depends on where in the body the self-antigens came from.

Well-known autoimmune diseases include type 1 diabetes, lupus, endometriosis and fibromyalgia. Some are fatal – Addison's disease, for example, killed Jane Austen. For a full list of autoimmune diseases, see the appendix to this book.

Autoimmune diseases

Autoimmune diseases, once considered rare, are now the second-highest cause of chronic illness in the United States and the top cause of morbidity (sickness) in American women. It's one of the top ten causes of death in women under the age of 65 and affects women 75 per cent more often than men. The US National Institutes of Health (NIH) estimates that around 23.5 million Americans suffer from an autoimmune disease, but this number pertains to only 24 of the 150-plus diseases (depending on who is counting) that fall under the umbrella of autoimmunity. It's believed the real figure is closer to 50 million (in a total population of 320 million) and growing. In addition, the NIH estimates that annual direct healthcare costs attributed to autoimmune diseases are approximately US$100 billion, far in excess of the annual cancer costs (US$57 billion) and heart disease and stroke costs (US$2.4 billion).

Studies have shown that the incidence of autoimmune disease is rising across the world, particularly since the 1950s. In Finland the incidence of type 1 diabetes has more than doubled within the last 30 years. Reality TV star Kim Kardashian recently revealed that like her mother, Kris Jenner, she suffers from the autoimmune condition psoriasis, while Venus Williams withdrew from the 2011 US Open citing the effects of Sjögren's syndrome. Popular Canadian model Winnie Harlow is known for having the auto-immune skin condition vitiligo that she developed at the age of four. In 2015, pop singer Selena Gomez announced that she had taken a break from public life to undergo chemotherapy treatment for lupus.

Autoimmune thyroid diseases are now rampant. Of note is the fact that the hypothyroid drug Synthroid is now the most commonly prescribed medication in the United States, with 21.6 million prescriptions issued from April 2014 to March 2015. Scientists have found that autoimmune thyroid disease frequently goes hand in hand with other autoimmune diseases, such as allergies, vitiligo, pernicious anaemia, multiple sclerosis, type 1 diabetes, and lupus. Both type 1 and type 2 diabetes (the second of which is not an autoimmune disease) are found in people suffering from rheuma-toid arthritis. It's thus worth noting that the rheumatoid arthritis drug Humira was the top-grossing drug in the United States during the same period, with sales of almost US$8.3 billion. Analysts have noted that the global market for autoimmune disease treatments is growing rapidly, particularly in the Asia–Pacific region, and will be worth US$15.97 billion by 2020. Dominant pharmaceutical industry players include Pfizer, Amgen and Abbott Laboratories.

According to Dr Noel R. Rose, chairman emeritus of the Scientific Advisory Board of the American Autoimmune Related Diseases Association (AARDA) and co-author (along with Australian Professor Ian R. Mackay) of the medical textbook *The Autoimmune Diseases*, autoimmune diseases are caused by a combination of several genes and the environment, and they can cluster in families. In December 2015, AARDA published highlights from a national conference on autoimmune diseases where decades of autoimmune research was distilled into a number of key points:

1. Autoimmune diseases have a genetic precursor that involves multiple genes. Two important gene families are involved in autoimmunity: the major histocompatibility complex (MHC) on chromosome 6, which determines what lymphocytes (immune cells) detect and how they react; and numerous other genes involved in regulating the immune system.

2. Genetics play only a small role in disease development – an outside trigger is required for the full disease to manifest itself. Autoimmune diseases develop in stages and may be detected in advance by predictive biomarkers (molecules in the blood that can be tested for), including elevated antibodies already circulating in a sufferer's system, despite a lack of disease symptoms.

3. Autoimmune diseases develop over time through a *constant* interaction between susceptible genes and environmental factors.
4. Autoimmune diseases primarily affect women of child-bearing age, and hormones may play a role. Autoimmunity is considered to be a major women's health issue.
5. Fatigue is a major feature of autoimmune diseases: six in ten sufferers note that fatigue would be the most debilitating aspect of their disease. Fatigue has been cited as a major cause of financial distress due to the patient's inability to maintain employment. In the United States, one in five sufferers had to claim disability because of their illness. (According to Noel Rose, fatigue is the main early symptom of most autoimmune disorders.)
6. Incidence of autoimmune diseases is increasing dramatically and is probably linked to environmental changes resulting from increasing industrialisation.
7. Damage to the microbiome (the bacterial population in the gut) is likely to be involved in disease development.
8. Environmental triggers include foods, drugs, biological agents, medical devices, tobacco smoke, UV light, pollution, stress, heavy metals such as mercury, and exposure to silica, beryllium and vinyl chloride (PVC) as well as pesticides.
9. Future avenues for preventing, diagnosing and treating autoimmune diseases will include Big Data, epigenetics (see page 93), greater understanding of T cell (see page 36) involvement, the role of diet, the role of the spleen, and technology.

Causes of autoimmune diseases

While the exact genetic and environmental combination for specific autoimmune diseases is unknown, researchers understand that certain pharmaceuticals can induce lupus in people, while environmental substances like silica, also known as silicon dioxide, can induce scleroderma. This is interesting considering a 2015 study indicated that nanoparticle silica, shown to interfere with DNA and the immune system, has been found in popular Australian foods including Old El Paso taco mix, Nestlé Coffee Mate, chicken salt, Roast Meat Gravy and Moccona Cappuccino. According to Friends of the Earth (FOE), which commissioned the study, these foods contained high levels of nanoparticles that have not been tested, labelled or approved for human consumption in Australia. FOE has since called for this issue to be urgently addressed by Food Standards Australia New Zealand, given the number of scientific studies that have raised health concerns involving the use of these nanoparticles in food.

The autoimmune summit experts also listed herbicides and pesticides as one of the non-infectious agents involved in disease development, and indeed we have faced decades of heavy global herbicide and pesticide use by agricultural companies. Given the world's bestselling herbicide glyphosate (Roundup) alongside malathion and diazinon were declared Class 2A carcinogens (i.e. probably carcinogenic to humans) by the IARC in March 2015, it's possible that further research may implicate agricultural products in other chronic health conditions.

In 2016, a 'Statement of Concern' was published in the journal *Environmental Health* noting that glyphosate was first sold to farmers in 1974, but its increased use in response to the emergence of glyphosate-resistant weeds and as a pre-harvest desiccant, and its widespread use in conjunction with genetically engineered soybeans, canola and alfalfa, means that its presence has become ubiquitous. In 1987 (before genetically engineered soybean and canola entered the market), between 2.72 and 3.62 million kilograms of glyphosate, representing 3.8 per cent of the total volume of herbicide being used, was applied by American farmers. In 1996, glyphosate-resistant crops started being grown commercially, and by 2008 this figure had risen to between 81.6 and 83.9 million kilograms or 53.5 per cent of the total herbicide volume and almost double the use of the broadleaf herbicide atrazine. The scientists note that the incidence of non-Hodgkin's lymphoma almost doubled during this time, and the number of severe birth defects has risen, particularly among farming communities. Glyphosate acts as an antibiotic and could alter the gastrointestinal microbiome, allowing overgrowth of pathogenic (disease-causing) bacterial species in affected populations.

More than 60 per cent of breads sold in the United Kingdom and the top fourteen brands of German beer have been found to contain traces of herbicides and pesticides, most frequently glyphosate, and US government testing revealed glyphosate residues in 90 per cent of 300 soybean samples (used in soymilk, infant formulas, sports drinks and animal feed), which means that consumers should potentially be concerned about this connection.

The deteriorating health of the younger generation has also become noticeable. The University of Bristol in the United Kingdom has been running the 'Children of the 90s' longitudinal study of children born in the 1990s and their parents. In early 2016, the research group published findings on what is considered to be the biggest study of chronic fatigue syndrome (CFS) in children to date. The study found that one in 50 British sixteen-year-olds is or has been affected by CFS, resulting in disrupted schooling, social isolation and even unjustified allegations by authorities of harm by parents. CFS, also known as myalgic encephalomyelitis, has been called yuppie flu in the past, but the researchers found that CFS sufferers tend to come from backgrounds with greater adversity, such as poor housing and financial stress, and the condition affects more girls than boys. In addition, many children and young people experience depression, behavioural and conduct disorders, anxiety, allergies, intolerances, immune system dysfunction and weight problems.

It's true that people are statistically more likely to have poor health if they are lower on the socioeconomic ladder but anecdotally it would seem that class and income make no difference to the new collection of 'physical breakdown' problems that seem to be at epidemic proportions. You are just as likely to have obesity, autoimmune conditions, CFS, depression, cancer, irritable bowel syndrome or metabolic syndrome issues in the leafy suburbs as you are in a mining town. Whatever is going on now could certainly be seen as a great equaliser. So what exactly is going on?

Big food

In recent times the finger of blame has been pointed at the fast- and processed-food industries. Their sophisticated advertising, often aimed at children, renders them the most obvious target of health activists. Yet lurking behind the often-blamed manufacturers and retailers of these foods sits an industrial-grade raw-material supply designed to feed millions cheaply. A cursory glance at the commodities index illustrates that alongside the energy and metals sector lie the foundations of our food supply.

Grains (wheat, barley, corn, rice), oilseeds (soybeans, canola, palm oil), other soft commodities (sugar, coffee, cocoa) and livestock (pigs and cattle), are traded in global markets daily, with prices rising and falling on the back of consumer demand. Grains, 'softs' and oilseeds are useful bulk commodities as they are easy to grow, store and transport, and in the last 50 years have played a major role in driving the growth of the processed-food industry. If we consider that sugar was first traded more than 200 years ago, and grains and oils followed almost 100 years later, we begin to appreciate that the genesis of the Western diet has always been rooted in the commodities trade.

While we are all familiar with the world's biggest food and beverage brands such as Unilever, Nestlé, Coca-Cola and General Mills, most of us would never have heard the names of four companies that controls the global bulk commodities supply. Known as the 'ABCDs' this group comprises Archer Daniels Midland, Bunge, Cargill and Louis Dreyfus.

The ABCDs have always been notoriously secretive, and since Louis Dreyfus and Cargill are family-owned businesses, it's difficult for researchers and analysts to obtain information about their activities. All of these companies are involved in producing, procuring, processing and delivering raw materials not just for use in our food, but for animal feed and biofuel.

Cargill is not only the largest of the 'Big 4' but also the largest privately owned company in the United States, with revenues of

US$120.4 billion. Founded in 1865, Cargill is a major commodities trader, buying and selling Western diet basics such as grain, corn, barley, sorghum, seed oils, sugar, soybeans, palm oil, cocoa, salt and oilseed, but its business interests are numerous, extending into meatpacking, finance and industrial products. In 2014, Cargill joined with Brazil's Copersucar to form the world's largest sugar trader. Brazil produces nearly half of the world's sugar, and the 50–50 deal enables Cargill to access Brazilian sugar without having to purchase sugar mills.

Archer Daniels Midland (ADM) had revenues of US$67.7 billion in 2015. Founded in 1902, it's the world's third-largest processor of wheat, corn, oilseed and cocoa, and is a major processor of soybeans, cottonseed, sunflower seeds, rapeseed and flaxseed. ADM grows and sells corn and sorghum, and has a 16 per cent share in Wilmar International, the largest palm oil trading company in the world.

Louis Dreyfus, founded in 1851 in France, is a family-owned business, generating US$64.7 billion in revenue in 2014. The firm trades in grains, oilseeds, coffee, sugar, wheat and rice, and is involved in processing soybeans for biofuel and animal feed. Louis Dreyfus is the oldest grain-trading company in Australia, having first opened an office in Melbourne in 1913.

Bunge was founded in 1818 and trades in grains, oilseeds, sugar and biofuel, and is the world's largest producer of soybean oil. The company generated US$57.8 billion in revenue in 2014. Bunge is the world's number one seller of seed oils to consumers.

The scale and scope of the ABCD firms' activities is substantial, given that they have pursued growth strategies based upon diversification of operations as well as vertical and horizontal integration.

Acquisitions, mergers and strategic partnerships are also common, such as Cargill Australia's purchase of the Australian Wheat Board in 2010. Not content to control the vast majority of the global bulk commodities trade, they are also understood to provide financing for raw material production; supply seeds, fertilisers and agrochemicals such as herbicides and pesticides; and own the storage facilities and transport mechanisms used to move their raw goods around the globe.

As originators of bulk commodities, the ABCD firms are in a position to work with farmers and producers to decide what to grow and how to grow it. The size, scale and volume of their operations provide them with immense leverage over market prices while acting as barriers against new market entrants. They focus their attention on generic products for use in processed food and animal feed, which enables them to fly under the radar of consumer angst surrounding the processed-food industry and the growing problem of agricultural chemical use.

Because they rarely own land, they are also distanced from issues concerning poverty-stricken small-scale farmers in developing nations, who while growing the raw materials that we consume on a daily basis, ironically make up the almost 900 million people who go to bed hungry each night. These companies are also rarely implicated in the environmental damage caused by agricultural production.

While the ABCD firms are quick to point out their role in feeding the world and alleviating global hunger, it's clear that their activities have contributed to broken food and health systems around the world. As distributors of the grains, sugar, salt, oilseeds, genetically modified soybeans and corn, cocoa and palm oil required to produce processed foods, they play a key role in the Western diet and in its now clear and present dangers.

The food manufacturers

The ABCD firms, and others like them, source the raw materials for the processed-food industry. It's up to food manufacturers to find innovative ways to turn cheap, tasteless carbohydrates such as flour and sugar, and disease-promoting seed oils into hugely profitable brands.

The process of buying low and selling high is referred to as 'value-adding' and was detailed in Michael Moss's 2013 exposé *Salt, Sugar, Fat: How the Food Giants Hooked Us*. Moss details the extraordinarily sophisticated chemistry employed by food manufacturers to turn otherwise bland and uninspiring raw materials into 'crave-able' snack and convenience foods and beverages that are big on 'mouthfeel' and boast 'bliss points' that hinge upon high levels of sugar, salt and fat. In addition to the food alchemy is a highly sophisticated marketing machine that exploits our deepest desires for comfort and a sense of belonging.

This magical combination enables the 'Big 10' food manufacturers to generate revenues of around US$1.1 billion per day. Such extraordinary market power affords these companies the ability to exert influence over the governments regulating the environments in which they operate.

According to Moss, at a meeting of industry heavyweights from Pillsbury, Kraft, Nabisco, General Mills, Coca-Cola, Mars, Procter & Gamble, Cargill and sugar giant Tate & Lyle in 1999, food-manufacturing heads were made aware of the role of their products in the growing epidemic of obesity, as well as the public's general inability to tolerate these foods physically. But the relentless drive for profit, growth and innovation resulted in the issue being given a mere cursory glance, and so what might have been the first real opportunity for change was lost in favour of the 'profits for shareholders' model. Given that food companies have known about the public-health ramifications of their products for a long time, it could be argued that diseases are now being imposed upon a largely unsuspecting society that has been left to pick up the financial and social costs of aberrant corporate behaviour.

Negative externalities

In the world of economics, unintended costs to society and the environment are referred to as 'negative externalities'. A negative externality occurs when an individual or a corporation makes a decision that has a negative impact on others but does not have to bear any of the costs of that decision. A case in point would be a processed-food company marketing high in sugar, seed oil and salt to people who may consequently become obese or develop high blood pressure, metabolic syndrome or type 2 diabetes. These conditions may lead to stroke, dialysis or amputations that in turn may result in physical disability, unemployment, poverty and family breakdown, the financial and social costs of which are picked up by the chronically diseased individual and the taxpayer. The corporation does not have to pay for the negative externalities generated by its products and marketing.

Sugar and fat taxes

One of the most discussed government-imposed remedies designed to mitigate the costs associated with obesity and food-related disease is the sugar and/or fat tax. While media debates about fat or sugar taxes mostly focus on the notion that a small increase in price to the consumer may result in people reducing their consumption, the main purpose of a junk food tax is to fund the increased healthcare costs associated with the negative externalities imposed on society as a result of the food industry's business practices. Food-industry lobbyists (who are employed to minimise regulation on behalf of their clients, even at the expense of wider public interest) typically fight any attempts to impose such taxes on the basis that they are 'unfair' and 'discriminatory' to business.

In January 2014, the Mexican government, concerned about the rapidly rising costs of treating diseases related to excess weight, imposed a tax of 1 Mexican peso per litre on sugary drinks. In a country where nearly three out of four adults are obese and 19 per cent of over-50s diagnosed with type 2 diabetes, the tax measure succeeded in creating public awareness of the health risks associated with sugary drinks and in changing consumer behaviour.

Sales of carbonated drinks sold by Mexico's biggest soft drink bottler, Coca-Cola FEMSA, fell by 6.4 per cent in the first half of 2014 compared to the first half of 2013, and the company blamed the fall on the sugar tax, bad weather and a weak economy. During the same period, sales of bottled water and milk increased.

One important issue that arose from the Mexican situation is that while US$1 billion was due to be raised via the tax in its first year, only US$100 million was allocated to install crucial drinking-water fountains in schools. Lack of access to clean drinking water is considered one of the key reasons Mexicans have relied on fizzy drinks. This highlights the need to make governments accountable for where any sugar or fat tax proceeds are ultimately allocated.

In November 2014 Berkeley in California followed suit, approving through a referendum the creation of a sugar tax that adds US$0.01 per calorie to soft drinks in an attempt to address rising rates of obesity and its associated costs. The electoral battle, known as Berkeley versus Big Soda, resulted in 75 per cent of voters favouring the tax, despite the industry spending US$3 million on a high-profile 'No' campaign. Given that 33 American cities had tried and failed to implement sugar taxes, the result in Berkeley was seen as a tipping point. Berkeley has long been known as a city at the forefront of social change, having ushered in the civil rights movement, the free speech movement, the Vietnam War protests, the disability rights movement, and smoking and Styrofoam bans. What happens in Berkeley is considered to be a barometer for what will happen elsewhere in three to five years.

In June 2016 Philadelphia City Council became the second location to vote for a 1.5 cent-per-fluid-ounce soda tax on sugary and diet drinks, with the funds to be allocated to preschools, community schools and park improvements. Some of the funds were also expected to go into the council's general fund.

In the United Kingdom, where 25 per cent of adults are now obese as opposed to only 3 per cent 40 years ago, Life Sciences Minister George Freeman recognised the issue of negative externalities generated by processed-food companies, noting that where certain products, such as sugar, confer costs on society, it might be reasonable to recoup those costs by taxing the firms that sell such products. Freeman's assertion was quickly rebuffed by a spokesperson for Prime Minister David Cameron, who expressed the government's tremendous reluctance to burden the 'hard-working people' with sugar taxes, which would likely increase the cost of their sugar-filled shopping baskets. Instead, noted the spokesperson, the government would continue with the tried and tested (and proven to fail) approach of 'working with industry' and various public-health bodies. In March 2016, Chancellor George Osborne announced a sugar tax on soft drinks to protect children's health and fund sport in primary schools. Interestingly, David Cameron, like Jeb Bush, is understood to follow the 200-year-old low carbohydrate Banting diet (see page 204) promoted by high-profile sports scientist Professor Tim Noakes, which eliminates added sugar, and prevents and can reverse many cases of type 2 diabetes.

The role of society

While processed food companies are routinely lambasted for their role in our current health crisis – and they are far from innocent bystanders – there are several other sides to the story, one of which includes the radical changes that have occurred in our society in a very short space of time. We lead increasingly busy and fast-paced lifestyles, forcing many of us to outsource the various apparatus of our lives, including the provision of our food. Longer working hours and the increase in the number of working mothers has also played a role in the demise of home cooking and family mealtimes. The proliferation of convenience-based processed, packaged and fast foods has become the enabler of our 'just in time' lives.

Children often start their school day fuelled by sugary breakfast cereals or cereal-based drinks high in refined carbohydrates and end the day with after-school junk-food snacks and a drive-through dinner. Well-meaning but time-poor parents fill lunchboxes with sugary, salty and seed-oil-rich snacks, inadvertently helping their kids become hooked on junk food and ultimately leading them down the road to future health problems. School canteens are not much better, many offering an assortment of processed foods and sugary drinks that, while attractive to children who don't know any better, offers little nutritional value to growing bodies that need nutrient density the most.

Uninformed or poor dietary decision-making by parents can come at a very frightening cost to the child. Careless and possibly uneducated behaviour by parents is now resulting in the removal of obese children from their parents in the United Kingdom. More than 70 obese children have been removed from their homes and placed in state care because of concerns about the long-term health impacts of a poor diet. Evidently, many parents were in denial, refusing to face up to the issue.

Perhaps there is a good reason governments need to strike first. A RAND Corporation report into kidney disease in the United States revealed that it's increasingly common for a dialysis practice to have first-degree type 2 diabetic relatives receiving dialysis in the same centre – for example, a mother, daughter and uncle might all receive dialysis treatment in the same centre at the same time, indicating that underlying health problems such as pre-diabetes are not being picked up and reversed through patient education or diet and lifestyle modification. Thus, the tragic consequence of poor diet and lifestyle is simply transferred from one generation to the next, and the opportunity to break the cycle of this terrible disease in families is lost.

Official nutritional advice

A fourth factor that has played a role in sending us down the road to an epidemic of food-related diseases is the rise of the 'diet expert'. The original diet expert was the United States Department of Agriculture (USDA), an organisation tasked with providing eating guidelines that, as it turns out, did a better job of reflecting economic and agricultural policies rather than nutritional science and public health.

One of the most illuminating books ever written on the political machinations and nutritional shenanigans that have historically lurked in the shadows of official dietary advice is *What to Eat: The Ten Things You Really Need to Know to Eat Well and Be Healthy* by Luise Light. Light was teaching at New York University in the late 1970s when she was approached by the USDA to develop a revised set of food guidelines to replace the Basic Four that had been around since 1956. With a background in public health, Light felt that it was important to devise a guide that better reflected chronic-disease prevention, which was a rapidly emerging problem even in the 1970s.

Light had been warned that 'heavy hitters' from the food industry would be monitoring her activities, while the agricultural-industry lobbyists had already made their presence known. Undaunted, Light pressed ahead and devised a plan based upon studies of health problems related to foods and nutrition, population diets and the latest nutritional science. In what was essentially the earliest incarnation of the famous food pyramid, the new food guide conceived by Light included:

- five to nine servings of fruits and vegetables as the foundation
- two to three servings of dairy
- 140–200 grams of protein such as red meat, poultry, fish, eggs, nuts or beans

- two to three servings of wholegrain bread, cereal, pasta or rice (two servings for women and men with sedentary lifestyles, three for teen boys and physically active men and women)
- 60 millilitres of 'good' fats, including olive oil, flaxseed oil and cold-pressed vegetable oils
- no more than 10 per cent of calories as sugar and no more than 30 per cent of calories from fats.

Light submitted her new food pyramid to the Secretary of Agriculture for review, but could scarcely have imagined the chain of events that was about to unfold. An amended version of the pyramid was returned to Light, with:

- six to eleven servings of grains (the prefix 'whole' had been omitted, giving the green light for people to consume refined grains or 'cheap carbos')
- three to four servings of dairy
- two to three servings of protein
- two to three servings of fruits and vegetables
- fats, oils and sweets suggested in vague terms to be 'used moderately'.

Alarmed at such a breathtaking distortion of her carefully calibrated guide, Light informed her supervisor, the agency director, that the changes would create an epidemic of obesity, diabetes and other diseases. The sheer volume of refined grains promoted by the new guide would not only add far too much refined carbohydrate (that the body would process like sugar) but would displace the health-promoting nutrient-dense foods, such as vegetables, fruits and protein.

In spite of Light's objections, the alterations stayed. In addition, the serving sizes were incorporated into the USDA's food stamps program and the school breakfast and lunch program in addition to any other feeding programs coordinated by the USDA. Congress ensured the serving sizes made it into legislation, meaning it would be against the law to fail to serve such quantities – a godsend for the merchants of grain. According to Light, the new rules meant that primary school children on the school lunch program would now consume eight daily servings of refined grains, while high school children would consume ten daily servings. This move delivered a US$350 million windfall to the wheat industry in America, and shifted public consumption habits towards a diet very high in refined carbohydrate.

Light's predictions eventually came to pass. In 1980, no US state had an obesity rate higher than 15 per cent. By 2014, obesity rates had risen to 29 per cent or higher in 28 US states, and today every US state sits above 20 per cent. Meanwhile, the chronic-disease problem highlighted in the famous 1977 'McGovern Report' became a chronic-disease epidemic.

THE MCGOVERN REPORT

This is the short name given to the 1977 report arising from what was officially called the United States Senate Select Committee on Nutrition and Human Needs, which was chaired by Senator George McGovern. The committee met between 1968 and 1977, initially to investigate concerns about hunger and malnutrition, which had been observed among poorer members of the population, particularly in southern states. In 1974, its scope was expanded to encompass overeating, and it began to focus on reformulating the government's 'healthy eating guidelines', in an effort to combat cardiovascular disease, type 2 diabetes and some cancers.

Since the *USDA Food Guide* system started in 1916, the public has been proffered nothing short of a baffling array of boxes, wheels, pyramids and plates from the diet experts, and yet the obesity and disease trajectory shows no sign of falling. Moreover, none of the advice has been as wildly off the mark as the epic-fail 'low-fat' recommendation based on a flawed cholesterol hypothesis. In 2015, the USDA all but conceded it had got that part wrong and now no longer warns people to avoid eggs, shellfish and other cholesterol-laden foods. Science writer and British Conservative peer Matt Ridley has suggested that there should be an 'inquiry into how the medical and scientific profession made such an epic blunder'.

In addition to promoting useful fictions around fat in the diet, the experts conveniently forgot to let us know that our new low-fat diets really meant we would be shifting to high-sugar diets – a move that has proven infinitely more dangerous than putting a knob of butter on our toast. The carbohydrate-heavy bottom layer of the pyramid, combined with sugar-spiked 'healthy' low-fat processed food is now being scrutinised for its contribution to our declining health. The excess sugar and carbohydrates it has introduced to our lives, combined with sedentary lifestyles, have promoted obesity and obesity-related chronic diseases.

In September 2015 the research arm of investment bank Credit Suisse published the findings of a year-long independent study into the low-fat message and the concomitant move towards high-carbohydrate diets (and increased omega-6 fat consumption), noting that the stance by US health officials created a health disaster of epic proportions. As the report points out, between 1971 and 2009, daily caloric intake has increased by just 12 per cent, but carbohydrate intake has risen from 215 to 280 grams per day – a 30 per cent increase. In the same period, protein intake increased 7 per cent, from 82 to 88 grams, and fat intake from 79 to 80.5 grams per day – just 2 per cent. In addition, Credit Suisse points out that consumption of corn has increased by 100 per cent, wheat by 21 per cent, seed oils by 89 per cent and sugar by 25 per cent. Credit Suisse noted that it expected a review of the neutral stance of health authorities on carbohydrates, given their role in the 4 per cent growth in metabolic syndrome, including type 2 diabetes and obesity.

In late 2015, the US Congress publicly noted that there was a serious issue with the scientific integrity of the *Dietary Guidelines for Americans*, and announced a Bill that would lead to a comprehensive review of the process behind developing the guidelines. Setting aside a US$1 million budget, the Bill gave the USDA 30 days to hire the National Academy of Medicine to conduct the review with the aim of better preventing chronic disease. In August 2016 the National Academy of Medicine announced its proposed review panel for this major taxpayer-funded effort, and the Nutrition Coalition, an advocate for nutrition policy (which comprised mostly doctors dealing with obesity-related diseases) that both preserves good health and fights nutrition related diseases, were quick to pounce. An analysis conducted by the Nutrition Coalition revealed that the panel was both unbalanced (38 per cent of the proposed members had no diet or nutrition experience) and was largely composed of government insiders, while the only obesity expert was also medical director of a line of diet products owned by Nestlé. In addition, the 2015 Dietary Guidelines Committee members participated in the selection process despite being told by Congress to recuse themselves from doing so.

It would seem that the diet experts have made a habit of running with both the sheep and the wolves, and professional reputations continue to diminish accordingly. One of the greatest grievances the public now has with the diet experts is the issue of industry funding and perceived conflicts of interest. Just as in Luise Light's era, it would seem that wherever nutritional research and policy are being made, Big Food and Big Ag still hover in the background.

Perhaps a glimmer of hope can be found at the Mayo Clinic. In recognition of the fact that 'everybody's different', it has developed a 'healthy weight pyramid' (dominated by vegetables and fruits) that can be tailored according to individual preference and needs. The not-for-profit organisation Oldways has developed a series of traditional eating guides, including an Asian diet pyramid, a Latin American diet pyramid, a Mediterranean diet pyramid. These all provide a useful counterpoint to the state-sanctioned, one-size-fits-all 'My Plate'.

In May 2015, the openly defiant Nutrition Australia, which is independent of the government, published its *Healthy Food Pyramid* with vegetables, fruits and legumes in the bottom, replacing the carbohydrate-heavy breads and cereals that have dominated the original pyramid's foundation for decades. Wholegrain carbohydrates fill the second section, while meat, dairy and nuts fill the third. No longer demonised, 'healthy fats' now fill the capstone of the pyramid. While this could be seen as a positive move away from the 'old wine in new bottles' tactic of the past, today's consumer is already mightily confused and advice like 'more fruits and vegetables' or even 'eat like great Grandma' is about all many of us can digest at this point. The vested interests behind the various incarnations of the dietary guidelines have created a bewildering mess, leaving us perplexed and increasingly deaf to the recommendations emanating from anybody who calls themselves a 'diet expert'.

What can we do?

The perfect storm of profit- and growth-driven bulk-commodity traders playing tag team with food manufacturers engaged in creating and marketing sugar, salt and fat-laden processed foods; societal changes favouring convenience over home cooking; and decades of corrupted, confusing and downright unhelpful food advice from those who clearly have something to gain means we have managed to sleepwalk into a situation from which we are finding it very difficult to extricate ourselves. Sadly, we have allowed a situation to develop in which the current generation of children are expected to live shorter lives than their parents. This is not due to the communicable diseases of our grandparents' era. Food will be the dominant disease vector, and the heart disease, cancer, metabolic syndrome and autoimmunity that stem from it will ensure that those lives are marred not just by disease but the inevitable suffering that goes with it.

A 'buy now, pay later, whatever's quickest, easiest and cheapest' attitude to food consumption might seem reasonable and justifiable at the time. But the problem, as many have discovered, is that eventually the chickens come home to roost. And if by that time you happen to be a 40-year-old working father with a stay-at-home wife, three children under ten and a mortgage, or a 30-year-old single mother supporting two children and struggling to pay the rent, those chickens might just herald the beginning of your worst nightmare. Daily pain and suffering, disability, depression, financial distress, family break-up, poverty and early death may be the harvest of seeds sown during the indestructible years of childhood and adolescence. Smart health decisions made during the developmental years can change the obesity, heart disease, cancer, autoimmunity and diabetes picture significantly.

3

The industry of sickness

He was a master business strategist, a ruthless and avowed monopolist and the most hated man in America. Having made his billions, he helped create a system of philanthropy involving such mammoth sums that he could dictate the terms upon which they were spent. And he had his sights set on sickness. But not even John D. Rockefeller (1839–1937) could have envisaged that in just over 100 short years three out of four of his countrymen and -women would be overweight or obese. Nor could he have foreseen that the malnutrition and communicable diseases that were the scourge of his era would make way for a raft of conditions leading to physical breakdown and rooted in too much energy-dense, seed-oil-saturated, nutrient-deficient food. He could not possibly have imagined that a tsunami of chronic disease would overwhelm the very system he helped create.

Rockefeller is not the name that springs to mind when you visit your local doctor, but he is the single biggest reason you will be prescribed pharmaceuticals rather than a low-carb or intermittent fasting diet for your metabolic syndrome symptoms. The story of how this happened goes back to the turn of the last century.

Rockefeller's medical revolution

You might be surprised to know that before 1910, 'orthodox' medical doctors in the United States unwittingly found themselves at the bottom of the healthcare food chain, at least as far as patients were concerned. Boldly referring to their own techniques as 'heroic', regular doctors routinely employed treatments such as profuse bloodletting, application of mercurous chloride or jalap to wounds, and the inducement of grotesque pus-filled blisters and violent vomiting.

In the event that a patient actually survived the bleeding, blistering, poisoning and purging, the doctor would administer an arsenic tonic and send them on their way with an invoice – and no doubt a three-month follow-up appointment. Indeed, 'Founding Father' Thomas Jefferson referred to doctors of his day as 'an inexperienced and presumptuous band of medical tyros let loose upon the world'. Increasingly fearful of the tendency of orthodox medicine to employ ever more distasteful, hazardous and futile 'therapies', safety-conscious patients preferred to take their chances with gentler treatments offered by herbalists.

So what happened in 1910 that would eventually result in the 'band of medical tyros' being elevated, unchallenged to the peak of public health? The Carnegie Foundation, John D. Rockefeller and a seeming nobody called Abraham Flexner. The almost universally loathed John D. Rockefeller of Standard Oil fame had developed an image problem. The oil monopolist was well known for his utter ruthlessness in business matters. He sabotaged competitors, infiltrated 'enemy' organisations with spies and crushed independent contractors via secret deals. He was also the subject of numerous investigating committees.

At this point, with a little help from a Baptist minister and public-relations counsellor called Frederick Taylor Gates, America's first billionaire and the richest man in history, a Baptist himself, expanded his efforts in what he called the 'difficult art of giving', setting his sights on what came to be known as 'strategic' philanthropy. An arrangement was created whereby money would be diverted from Rockefeller and his industrialist friends and used to create social change.

In earlier years, Rockefeller had channelled funds into teaching schools and educational research, which meant he could not only buy influence and dominate the education sector, but could also shape the direction of the entire field. He and Gates set up the General Education Board in 1902, which he funded with millions to be directed into higher education institutions all over America, and the creation of a teacher-training college for African Americans, and high schools and farming education in the southern states.

As a result, education turned away from being the preserve of the elites and was progressively opened up to more and more Americans. In the democratisation process, education turned away from its classical humanities base towards the modern science-based system we still have today. Some have suggested that this was a deliberate move to turn out minimally educated mass workforces that would provide labour to 'robber baron' industries, rather than informed and enlightened humans capable of challenging 'the system' Rockefeller had played a large role in creating. Others would suggest that it had the opposite effect. Whatever the outcome, having achieved vast changes in the education sector, Rockefeller, with the help of Gates and an educator by the name of Abraham Flexner, was about to do the same thing with human health.

Flexner was a primary schoolteacher from Kentucky and an educational researcher at the Carnegie Foundation, which oversaw the philanthropy of industrialist Andrew Carnegie. While at the Carnegie Foundation, Flexner was asked to visit more than 155 medical schools in the United States and Canada over the space of eighteen months and assess the current educational standards and overall quality of the schools. Flexner also visited medical schools in England, Scotland, Germany and Austria. In 1910, the Carnegie Foundation published his final report, 'Medical education in the United States', commonly known as 'The Flexner report of 1910'.

Before the report was published, Flexner had been summoned by Gates to have lunch. Gates was very interested in the German medical schools, which placed a heavy emphasis on scientific research, and was strongly opposed to the homeopathy favoured not just by Rockefeller himself (who incidentally lived to almost 98 years old) but the wealthy and educated classes in general. Gates offered to make a donation of US$1 million, a huge sum in 1910, for the purpose of developing medical education in the United States, and this money was eventually received in 1913 by his German-oriented alma mater, Johns Hopkins University.

Flexner left the Carnegie Foundation the same year and joined the Rockefeller-controlled General Education Board to 'direct the allocation of Rockefeller millions to the development of *chemically oriented medicine* in the United States'. Between 1913 and 1960, the General Education Board gave a total of US$96 million to medical schools that exclusively used chemicals and surgery. In the allocation of these funds, Gates was adamant 'that medicine must serve capitalist society and be controlled . . . by capitalist foundations and capitalist universities'. Sympathetic media connections facilitated the public demonisation of all other healthcare competition to this new medical model, and 'voices calling for an ethos of patient welfare were silenced'.

The General Education Board also allocated huge sums to the Gates-controlled Rockefeller Institute for Medical Research, which was initially run by Abraham Flexner's pathologist brother, Simon. Under Simon's leadership the institute focused its resources on chemistry, biology, pathology, bacteriology, physiology, pharmacology and experimental surgery. Gates genuinely believed that science and technology could solve society's ills and that medicalising social problems – such as poor health or malnutrition – by utilising chemical solutions was the best way forward.

The influence on modern medicine of the Rockefellers, the Carnegies, the Flexner brothers and Frederick Taylor Gates cannot be underestimated. As a result of the Flexner Report, the German system of science-based medicine was catapulted into the ascendancy. The industry reforms, which were by no means all bad, included strict licensing arrangements and an end of 'for-profit' medical schools, standardised basic care, advances in surgery, improved hygiene, evidence-based medicine, vastly better training for doctors, shared knowledge, and well-equipped hospitals and laboratories. Jefferson's lancet-wielding 'tyros' were finally reined in, and through science were given discipline, direction, legitimacy, status, authority and power.

The Johns Hopkins template for medical training can now be seen in hospitals across the globe. The pharmaceutical industry has also flourished. Today, the global revenue generated by the pharmaceutical sector is in the vicinity of US$1 trillion, up from US$390 billion in 2001 and a mere US$6 billion in 1980, when the obesity epidemic could be said to have commenced. Rockefeller, the world's richest man, sure was on to something. (Although, as we will see in Chapter 9, the growth of the pharmaceutical industry is finally starting to slow.)

Little more than 100 years after the Flexner Report was published, a paradox has emerged. How can we be so medically and scientifically enlightened and simultaneously be facing a world-wide epidemic of chronic disease? How can we be so well placed to understand and prevent chronic disease, yet so glaringly incapable of doing so? Did the massive investment in and subsequent swing towards the reactive, chemically based and capitalist model of 'health care' become so culturally entrenched that it has rendered the entire field hopelessly ill-equipped to respond meaningfully in an era where diet, lifestyle and environmental factors have become the most dominant disease vectors? Can a profit-seeking, chemical model of medicine really save us from the harms inflicted by profit-seeking processed-food companies?

Profit at any cost

During my years working in the corporate world, I was unquestionably of the mind that the role of a business was to deliver profit and shareholder value to the 'true owners' of the company, the shareholders. End of story. How I came upon this view, I can't really recall. It just seemed that everybody was singing from the same hymn sheet and 'profit and shareholder value' was the universally agreed tune.

While the debate about corporate purpose has raged for decades, the most prominent voice in the shareholder value argument has been Milton Friedman, economist and teacher at the Chicago School of Economics and 1976 Nobel Prize winner for Economics. In 1970, the *New York Times Magazine* published an article by Friedman titled 'The social responsibility of business is to increase its profits' in which he slammed long-held ideas that businesses should maintain a social conscience, provide employment, avoid pollution or eliminate discrimination, referring to such behaviours as 'unadulterated socialism'.

In his article, Friedman stated as more or less fact that business in general cannot be said to have responsibilities. A corporate executive, however, was the exception to this rule: 'A corporate executive is an employee of the owners of the business [i.e. the shareholders] . . . his primary responsibility is to them'. Friedman, however, misled his readers on two fronts. First, shareholders do not legally own a corporation, they merely hold shares in it; and secondly, corporate executives are legally employed by the corporation, not by its shareholders.

Based on Friedman's flawed concept, any humanitarian feelings a corporate executive might harbour – ensuring, for example, that customers are happy with products or services; or that junk foods, agricultural chemicals, pharmaceuticals or foods containing GMOs are proven unquestionably safe before being unleashed on the public – would be clearly misguided, bordering on 'socialist'.

Friedman's article also makes explicit the strict profit motive of the corporation, insisting that a business has but a single social responsibility: 'to use its resources and engage in activities designed to increase its profits [i.e. maximise shareholder value]' as long as it plays by the rules. This is known in business as the shareholder primacy view.

Somewhere along the way, however, Friedman's 'idea' with regard to shareholder value and increasing profits seems to have morphed into unquestioned belief in a connection between profit and corporate law. But Friedman was an economist – not a corporate lawyer. In her book *The Shareholder Value Myth*, distinguished professor of corporate and business law at Cornell School of Law, Lynn Stout, explains that because the shareholder primacy *idea* is taught to students in top business schools, the philosophy has permeated the business world as an unchallenged default position.

Stout notes in her book that during her time as a law student in the 1980s, her teachers taught her that shareholders 'own' corporations and that corporate purpose was to 'maximise shareholder value'. It wasn't until many years later that Stout began to question her own conditioning. I'm sure I too did my own fair share of handwringing about 'the shareholders' to various clients over the years, until I realised that nobody in business I questioned on the subject could clearly articulate what shareholder value actually was. It would seem that Lynn Stout and I were both 'slaves to some defunct economist', as John Maynard Keynes would have said.

According to Stout, a key problem with the shareholder value position is that it's not supported by the conventions of American corporate law, nor is it consistent with the true economic structure of a typical business corporation. In addition, the idea of placing shareholders first is not supported by the majority of empirical evidence on what makes corporations and economies work. When visiting Australia in 2011, Stout stated: 'I'm saying this as a law professor. This is a legal fact. There is no legal duty to maximise shareholder value . . . you won't find it in US law.'

And yet several decades have now passed with corporations beholden to what iconic CEO Jack Welch called 'the dumbest idea in the world'. According to Stout, shareholder value ideology has resulted in an epidemic of short-termism, in which corporate managers have become fixated on short-term earnings at the expense of long-term performance. In addition, a focus on shareholders has discouraged investment and innovation, and indeed 'harms employees, customers, and communities; and causes companies to indulge in reckless, sociopathic, and socially irresponsible behaviours'. Moreover, it essentially threatens the overall welfare of the wider community, including staff, consumers and investors themselves.

A cursory glance across the corporate landscape indeed throws up a history of high-profile US disasters stemming from precisely the behaviours Stout describes – the collapse of Enron, BP's Deepwater Horizon oil spill, the *Exxon Valdez* oil spill, Countrywide's subprime loans, the Citibank collapse, the WorldCom scandal and others. At the extreme end of shareholder value thinking lies the extraordinary case of former hedge fund executive Martin Shkreli, who in his new job as biotech boss raised the price of the drug Daraprim required by HIV patients among others to treat toxoplasmosis from US$1130 to US$63,000 per treatment. Shkreli described the price hike as an example of good business decision-making, noting that shareholders expected him to generate as much profit as possible – a business approach that Shkreli dismissed quite simply as the 'ugly, dirty truth'.

Like me, Lynn Stout recognises the important role of big business and the peace, prosperity and opportunity it's capable of providing. But she argues for new thinking akin to a 'doing well by doing good' model that generates long-term growth for both investors and factors in society and the environment.

Stout's assessment is not to suggest shareholders have no rights, but quite the contrary. The tiny US state of Delaware is where the majority of Fortune 500 firms such as Cargill, McDonald's, Coca-Cola, Merck and Co., Novartis, GlaxoSmithKline, Apple and Google are domiciled. These companies prefer Delaware because of its 'favourable' corporate taxes, 'sympathetic' regulatory environment, 'modern' approach to corporate law, and expertly trained, astute and highly respected legal minds. Delaware has a unique court called the Court of Chancery that rules on corporate law disputes without juries.

The Honourable Leo E. Strine Jnr, a former acting chancellor of the Delaware Court of Chancery, is now chief justice of the Delaware Supreme Court. Chief Justice Strine has highlighted a number of 'inconvenient truths' with respect to challenging notions of shareholder primacy – namely that in American corporate law, shareholders are the only group in a position to:

- elect directors
- vote on corporate transactions
- charter amendments

- legally enforce the corporation's compliance with corporate law
- legally enforce the director's compliance with their fiduciary duties.

This allocation of power, he notes, has a powerful effect on how directors govern for-profit corporations. Naturally, when only one constituency is in the position to displace the board, 'it is likely that the interests of that constituency will be given primacy'. Strine, however, concedes, 'When the pressure to deliver profits becomes ... more intense, the rules of the game become even more important.'

The health system

While Stout's clarification of the law and Strine's practical realities help explain why corporations often behave in a counterintuitive fashion with regard to communities, public health and the environment, such insights expose the rock and the hard place between which corporate executives find themselves stuck. Both the bulk-commodity and processed-food industries, in order to deliver shareholder value (profit) under the shareholder primacy model must rely on increased sales and expanding markets for their respective products. Increased sales and expanded markets will by default result in excessive negative externalities – in other words, more chronically sick people and a significant societal burden.

The tab for the 'chronic diseasing' of society (as a socially destructive negative externality of the food industry) must inevitably be picked up by the taxpayer via the 'health sector', which is composed of three major components:

1. doctors and hospitals
2. health insurance companies
3. pharmaceutical companies.

Of these, the pharmaceutical sector unquestionably (and perhaps unquestioningly) favours the shareholder primacy view.

Doctors and hospitals

Doctors are, for the most part, the primary interface between patients (consumers) and hospitals, health insurance companies and pharmaceutical companies. They sit at the retail end of the sickness experience: meeting patients, diagnosing conditions, treating ailments, facilitating surgery, and providing ongoing treatment products and services as well as facilitating hospital care. While diagnostics form a large part of modern-day medicine, today's doctor must handle disease largely via the chemically oriented, capitalist-based medical model. This becomes a problem when 'lifestyle diseases' or perhaps 'negative externality diseases' are swamping the system.

Many doctors appear to pay little attention to diet and nutrition, and this could be for a number of reasons: limited time to spend with patients, patient attitude, or an expectation that health problems should be addressed in the near term, leading to an over reliance on medication. Perhaps another contributing factor is that nutrition education appears to be limited in many medical schools. A 2010 survey conducted in the United States revealed that of 109 schools targeted, 103 required some form of nutrition education, but only 26 of them required a dedicated nutrition course. Overall, US medical students received 19.6 contact hours or two and a half days of nutrition instruction during their six years in medical school.

While the US National Academy of Sciences sets a minimum of 25 hours of nutritional education for American trainee doctors, only 27 per cent of the 105 schools that answered this question met this requirement in 2010, a drop from 38 per cent in 2004. Given that the majority of hospital admissions stem from poor diet and lifestyle, the current pharmaceutical emphasis in medical training ultimately leaves doctors in an increasingly untenable position akin to taking a knife to a gunfight. Indeed, this very conundrum was noted by Dr Beverly Winikoff, then of the Rockefeller Foundation, in her January 1977 statement to the press regarding the McGovern Dietary Goals for the United States: 'Appropriate public education must emphasise the unfortunate but clear limitations of current medical practice in curing the common killer diseases.'

One doctor who recognised the superiority of diet over drugs in returning his patients to health was the famous human rights activist and pioneer of the community health centre movement in the United States Dr H. Jack Geiger. In 1967, Geiger created the first US community health centre in poverty-stricken Mound Bayou, Mississippi. The health centre was funded by the Office of Economic Opportunity as part of the US government's wildly unsuccessful 'war on poverty'. While Geiger's clinic provided standard medical services, he also understood that social determinants such as malnutrition, environmental issues, poverty and unemployment underpinned the health of the individual and community. While poverty, environmental issues and unemployment were harder problems to fix, malnutrition was easily addressed via access to nutritious food. Healthy individuals could then improve their chances of employment and lift themselves out of the poverty trap.

With this in mind, Geiger allocated funds from the Office of Economic Opportunity for the purpose of prescribing food for his patients. These prescriptions would be filled by the local supermarket and paid for by the clinic's pharmacy. When the Office of Economic Opportunity was alerted to Dr Geiger's nutrition scheme, various bureaucrats were dispatched to Mississippi to demand he use standard medical therapies – in other words, pharmaceuticals. Geiger is famously reputed to have replied, 'The last time we looked in the [Physician's Desk Reference] the specific therapy for malnutrition was food.'

Almost 50 years later, not much has changed. In my experience and anecdotally, discussions around possible dietary responses to autoimmunity, type 2 diabetes reversal, gastrointestinal problems, mood and behavioural problems and other chronic disease symptoms are not a major feature of health management strategies. Doctors are trained under the pharmaceutical model, the vast majority of medical research is funded and conducted with a view to developing a chemical response to illness and, as the 2010 nutrition survey demonstrated, this is unlikely to change any time soon. This unfortunate situation only compounds the negative externalities generated via the food chain.

A further inadequacy of our health system is that doctors exist within the silos of their specialisation and rarely collaborate across disciplines. For example, a patient may primarily suffer from autoimmunity brought on by a combination of their genetics and their unique environment, but the manifestations of their condition may span their thyroid, skin, gastrointestinal tract and joints. These problems inevitably require an ensemble of specialists (endocrinologist, dermatologist, gastroenterologist and rheumatologist) all operating independently of each other and relying on differing protocols. The problem of the lack of integration between medical specialisations may eventually be solved, however, as a by-product of the explosion of autoimmune diseases in the West.

Professor Yehuda Shoenfeld, head of Israel's Zabludowicz Center of Autoimmune Diseases, founder and editor of the *Israel Medical Association Journal*, author of *The Mosaic of Autoimmunity* and the textbook *Autoantibodies*, and author of more than 1000 research papers on autoimmunity and rheumatology, proposed the introduction of the world's newest doctor, the multidisciplinarily trained 'autoimmunologist', as a means of providing better care and reducing costs for patients suffering from conditions that span multiple tissues and organs.

A final reason our current pharmaceutical-based medical model cannot deal with the epidemic of food-based and environmental diseases is that preventative care does not generate revenue for the doctors, hospitals and corporations that profit from sickness. Healthy diets composed of nutrient-dense, chemical-free foods, regular exercise and the 'de-medicalisation' of preventative care do not make money for the tiny number of individuals and investors for whom an increasingly sick and drug-dependent society is a financial imperative. In addition, the fee-for-'service' rather than fee-for-'outcome' model ensures that this will not change any time soon.

People usually become doctors because they want to help people. They want to use their skills to assist the unwell and then send them back into the world to their families, jobs and lives. But the current tsunami of diet and lifestyle diseases leaves doctors in the position of paddling with both arms tied behind their back. Pharmaceuticals and surgery can only mitigate symptoms and do not address the underlying issues causing the tsunami. Until these are addressed, the waves will keep coming and the costs, both financial and social, will keep rising. Rich and poor alike will continue to pay for this crisis with their taxes and eventually their lives.

Health insurance companies

The health insurance industry is dominated by large firms, some of which are 'not-for-profit' and plough their earnings back into member services, while others are for-profit and arguably operate under the shareholder primacy model. These firms generate income through premiums, 'add-ons' and taxes. Irrespective of profit motives, the business model relies on maintaining an optimal ratio between income from healthy policyholders, who pay premiums yet rarely or never claim, and less healthy policyholders, who pay premiums yet make more regular claims. Like governments, they are also keen to keep costs such as those for hospital stays and medications to a minimum. For this reason, health insurance companies have a vested interest in a healthy population to offset costs associated with high-risk policyholders.

To this end, it's common for health insurance companies to promote healthy living and to educate the public regarding preventative health measures such as maintaining healthy weight and giving up smoking. For example GMHBA offers a Chronic Disease Management Plan, a Strong Knees Program and a Bowel Cancer Risk Identification Program, while BUPA provides Living Well programs such as gym memberships, yoga and Pilates courses, and weight management programs. Health insurance companies are mindful of what people need to be healthy and not get sick in the first place.

Pharmaceutical companies

To a large degree, the financial goal of the health insurance industry sits diametrically at odds with that of the pharmaceutical industry, as the first makes money from the healthy, while the second makes money from the sick.

Pharmaceutical companies have relied heavily on the vertically integrated, patent-protected blockbuster drug strategy for decades, controlling everything from the research laboratories and manufacturing plants to the large, sophisticated and expensive sales and marketing teams that have traditionally targeted doctors in their efforts to reach consumers. In recent years, however, this model started to wobble, as product pipelines waned, top-selling products went off patent and generic medications flooded the market, forcing pharmaceutical companies to adapt or incur the wrath of analysts and shareholders. Tactics included trimming costs and product lines, diversification into consumer products and over-the-counter items such as vitamins, and securing new markets in developing nations and newly Westernised countries hit hard by Western diseases.

Pharmaceutical companies have also faced numerous high-profile product-safety scandals that have served to erode public trust in both the companies and their products. There is today growing public concern about the level of influence the pharmaceutical industry exerts over the medical profession, medical research and training of young doctors. Consumers have also become frustrated with the hit-and-miss, trial-and-error nature of health care, where debilitating side effects from medications are sometimes blamed on the patient, ignored or treated with yet another drug. It's becoming painfully apparent that very few people ever seem to actually get better in the long run. A strategy of 'managing symptoms' in an increasingly chronically-diseased world has become a recipe for financial and social disaster.

Doing well by doing good

Will this situation continue to spiral out of control? Or will a combination of unforeseen but rapidly escalating forces diminish the previously unchallenged domination of consumer health by the chemically oriented capitalist model? Could this usher in a new era of health care based upon supporting and promoting the common health rather than stripping the common wealth?

While it's hard to say exactly what the outcome may be, the pressing need for the industry of sickness to recalibrate itself into an industry of genuine health is becoming increasingly apparent. The costs to taxpayers and societies of a business-as-usual, pill-for-every-ill mentality are simply too high. It's likely that the successful health insurance company of the future will be one that understands today's healthcare consumer and determines innovative ways to reward customers, financially or otherwise, for adhering to desired health behaviours. Rewarding healthcare consumers for measurably improving and sustaining their personal healthcare metrics would lead to lower costs for consumers, governments, employers and health insurance firms.

Profit-seeking companies will always seek profit, and we would be naïve to believe this will change anytime soon. The way they make profit, however, is ripe for change. In 2014, the Aspen Institute's Business and Society Program reopened the question of corporate purpose, exploring the beliefs of investors, corporate leaders and scholars from the US business world. When participants were asked to discuss both sides of the shareholder primacy debate, it turned out that both corporate executives and institutional investors personally felt that the role of the corporation was to serve customers' interests, while academics felt the role was to serve shareholders' interests, reiterating the view Lynn Stout claims is prevalent in business schools.

While the attitudes may demonstrate a small shift away from the shareholder primacy model, it shows that executives are starting to rethink the purpose of the corporation in modern society in what may be the green shoots of a 'doing well by doing good' post-Friedman era. Perhaps best exemplifying this shift is the rise of the benefit corporation, commonly known as the B corp. Benefit corporations are 'for-profit' companies that have voluntarily signed up to be part of a movement that redefines corporate success by creating businesses that have a positive impact on the world. Benefit corporations pledge to consider the needs of all stakeholders of a business, including employees, communities and shareholders, an ethos that flies in the face of that underpinning the shareholder primacy model. More than 1000 businesses around the world have joined the movement, including 77 Australian companies – and the momentum is growing. There are even increasing numbers of visionary and values-driven executives who have a strong preference for selling their skills only to companies that define themselves as benefit corporations, and these numbers will undoubtedly increase as more companies come on line.

Benefit corporation statutes for both private and public companies have now been adopted by the District of Columbia in addition to nineteen US states, including Delaware, home of many of the Fortune 500. In a 2014 article that appeared in the *Harvard Business Law Review*, Chief Justice Leo Strine described the B corp effort as a practical, real-world solution to the 'profit at any cost' problems raised by Lynn Stout, noting that the movement was in his view 'refreshing'. Strine suggests that getting this model right is a work in progress, but that its robustness and ability to endure and thrive under full market conditions will only be revealed with time.

Now that the seeds to the benefit corporation have been sown, the movement could ultimately yield enterprises that are in a position to break new ground, enabling ethical entrepreneurs to build large-scale food-and-health-related businesses that abide by the 'doing well by doing good' philosophy. Such businesses may include:

- health insurance companies that provide discounted health insurance to demonstrably health-conscious consumers
- 'food as healthcare' companies
- clean, green, organic farming businesses that sell direct to the consumer or supply other businesses that will in turn create value-added health products
- restaurant and café chains and meal-delivery businesses that sell ethically and locally sourced, clean and healthy products to local communities
- integrated diet, exercise and wellness gymnasium chains ('wellnasiums'!)
- nutritional supplement companies that sell green, clean prebiotics, probiotics, vitamins and minerals

- medical centres with an emphasis on disease prevention through long-term doctor–consumer collaborations regarding diet and lifestyle changes rather than patriarchy and pills
- health and wellness travel companies
- health and wellness resorts accessible to mainstream consumers at a fair-minded cost
- healthy workplace vending machine operators along the same lines as LeanBox
- vegan mixed retail stores like Europe's Veganz chain
- clean label technology companies.

The industry of sickness is crude, unethical, unsustainable and reflects not just the utter greed and ruthlessness of the warped Friedman model but the gulf between the Rockefeller ideology spawned more than 100 years ago and the challenges of responding to an environment that is making us sick today.

The new game in town will be played by health professionals who understand the key drivers of the current health crisis and are determined to reclaim their true heritage, stated in Hippocrates' original oath: 'with regard to healing the sick, I will devise and order for them the best diet . . . and I will take care that they suffer no hurt or damage'. In addition, enlightened and values-driven entrepreneurs will build capacity for the rapidly growing educated, intelligent and switched-on consumers who have simply had enough of watching one of the greatest human tragedies in the history of the human race unfold before them.

4

Not everything is genetic

Among the thousands of researchers to grace the Rockefeller Institute, one lone scientist was more interested in the cause than the cure. René Dubos was a pioneering microbiologist, experimental pathologist, Pulitzer Prize–winning writer and environmentalist. As a trained agronomist (agricultural plant scientist), he was most noted for his groundbreaking research on antibacterial substances, which led to the development of the first antibiotics. In later years he wrote extensively on the mechanisms of tuberculosis (the disease that so ravaged Weston Price's indigenous groups), pneumonia and adaptive immunity, as well as susceptibility and resistance to infection. His detailed knowledge of pathogens (disease-causing organisms) led him in 1942 to predict that bacteria would eventually become resistant to antibiotics, an unfortunate situation that has now come to pass.

Dubos's research gave him unique insight into the environmental causes of disease, and in the late 1950s he was already 'pointing out the futility of relying on medicine to cure the ills created by social and physical environments'. His work in tuberculosis led him to conduct studies on 'the influence of metabolic factors, nutrition and environmental stresses on host resistance to various infectious diseases'. Decades ahead of his time, this extraordinary leading-edge thinker was already focusing his research on the impact of environmental factors on the composition of normal gastrointestinal flora (gut bacteria, collectively known as the microbiome or microbiota) and its consequences in terms of the host's development and resistance to disease.

In recent years, it has been confirmed that the gut microbiota plays many important physiological roles, such as 'digestion, metabolism, extraction of nutrients, synthesis of vitamins, prevention [of] colonisation by pathogens and immunomodulation'. Indeed, environmental factors such as the Western diet, antibiotics, caesarean birth and lack of breastfeeding have already been implicated in the development of a lower and less diverse intestinal bacteria count in humans, which has the potential to lead to allergies and numerous chronic diseases.

In his professional life, René Dubos was the recipient of no less than 28 awards and memberships and 41 honorary degrees. Dubos also published many books, including *The White Plague: Tuberculosis, Man and Society* (1952), in which he expounded his theory that susceptibility to infection was connected to an altered environment; *The Dreams of Reason: Science and Utopias* (1961), in which he challenged the ability of science to eliminate disease; and *Man Adapting* (1965), which put forward the idea that health or disease are an adaptive response to environmental challenges.

Dubos passed away on his eighty-first birthday in 1982, but his ideas are entering a renaissance period as science makes rapid breakthroughs not just in human genetics and epigenetics (changes in gene expression due to environmental factors) but also that of our human microbiome. In addition, the field of nutrigenomics is merging cutting-edge nutritional research with genomics (gene sequencing) to better understand how common dietary inputs affect health by altering the structure or expression of our genes. While Dubos did not live to see the commencement of the Human Genome Project in 1990, he could scarcely have imagined just how much scientific evidence would eventually be found to support his conceptual frameworks.

The discovery of DNA's role in genetics

At one point along my own journey with chronic disease, I remember being told by a doctor that my situation 'was genetic': it was 'destiny' and I should just accept my fate – which I did. Unfortunately, many sick or unhealthy people are given the same disempowering information – they are obese because they have the FTO or 'fat gene', depressed because they have the 'depression gene', developed cancer because they have the 'cancer gene' or even vote left of centre because they have the 'liberal gene' – and yet the scientific evidence does not support the idea that, apart from rare cases, our genes are our destiny. Despite studying the genes of thousands of individuals, researchers have found that heritability makes only a modest contribution to most diseases.

In fact, the rapid spread of chronic diseases throughout countries and cultures around the globe in a very short space of time would indicate that genetic changes are unlikely to be responsible. But that is not to say that genes don't matter, because they clearly play a role in susceptibility to disease.

To understand exactly where our genes enter the chronic-disease picture, we need to go back in time – once again to the Rockefeller Institute. I can't help but wonder if René Dubos, on his likely campus strolls or cafeteria visits, ever crossed paths with fellow scientists Oswald T. Avery, Maclyn McCarty or Colin MacLeod. If he did, we might only imagine the debate that may have taken place. In 1944, Avery, McCarty and McLeod demonstrated that deoxyribonucleic acid (DNA) in bacteria carried inherited genetic information, a breakthrough that heralded the beginnings of DNA research and the eventual realisation that DNA is in fact the universal language of life.

In 1948, two-time Nobel Prize–winning chemist and biochemist Linus Pauling discovered that some proteins take the shape of an alpha helix – spiralled like a coil. In 1953, Pauling published a paper proposing a triple helical structure for DNA, which is not a protein but had the potential to form a similar structure. Two Cambridge researchers, Francis Crick and James Watson, who had also developed a theory based on a triple helical structure, were intrigued by Pauling's ideas. The triple helical concept, however, turned out to be slightly off the mark.

One year earlier, in 1952, British DNA researcher Raymond Gosling, working under Rosalind Franklin, produced an X-ray diffraction photo of a DNA molecule. The famous 'photograph 51' clearly showed an 'X' shape in the middle of the molecule, indicating that it was a twin helical structure. Yet another DNA researcher, Erwin Chargaff, had shown in 1950 that the four bases that were part of the DNA structure – adenine, thymine, guanine and cytosine – 'paired' in the same ratios, for example the amount of adenine equals that of thymine and guanine equals cytosine, a discovery known as Chargaff's rules. The base pairs are usually abbreviated to G, A, T and C (the title of the Hollywood film *GATTACA*, a story that features a dystopian future in which people's genes determine their place in society, comes from a combination of these abbreviations). When Gosling and Franklin's diffraction studies on DNA were combined with Chargaff's rules, it became apparent that the base pairs held the double helix structure of DNA together.

By combining the knowledge of the double helix and base pairing, Francis Crick and James Watson were able to determine that the base pairs fitted together like rungs on a twisted ladder. Watson and Crick published their paper titled 'Molecular structure of nucleic acids – a structure for deoxyribose nucleic acid' in *Nature* in April 1953. The breakthrough provided an understanding of how genetic material was passed from one generation to the next. Today the famous image of the double helix is universally recognised. In 1962, Watson, Crick and Rosalind Franklin's research partner Maurice Wilkins won the Nobel Prize for discovering DNA. As Franklin had died from cancer several years earlier, she did not receive the prize and in fact was never nominated. The contributions of Raymond Gosling, Oswald T. Avery and Erwin Chargaff towards the discovery of DNA were also overlooked by the Nobel Prize committee.

The human genome

In 1990, almost 30 years later, the Human Genome Project (HGP) was announced with the goal of identifying and sequencing all 3 billion base pairs in the human genome, ostensibly to identify the genetic roots of illness and disease such as cancer and diabetes. The idea was simple – that targeted treatments for disease could be developed based on genetic variants. By 2001, Dr Francis Collins, the director of the National Human Genome Research Institute, hailed the discoveries as providing a virtual shop manual that would offer healthcare providers the chance to treat, prevent and cure disease. After spending billions of dollars of both public and private money, the HGP was declared finished in April 2003, well ahead of schedule.

While the global chronic-disease burden has and will continue to mount despite the unveiling of the 'shop manual', it would appear that cracking the human genome was more akin to opening a can of worms that has resulted in more questions than answers. None of these is more perplexing, particularly where chronic disease is concerned, than the case of 'missing heritability'.

The human body is made of 70–100 trillion cells, each of which must contribute to the seven requirements for life: movement, reproduction, sensitivity, growth, respiration, excretion and nutrition in order to survive and produce the chemistry necessary to maintain the life of the overall organism – you! At the centre of most of these cells is the nucleus, and housed inside the nucleus are two sets of genes – one from your mother and one from your father.

DNA works by providing the instructions – as a code using combinations of the four bases (G, A, T, C) – that a cell needs to make proteins. Within a living organism, proteins provide basic structure as well as catalyse all the cellular processes that produce other vital structural and metabolic components. The Human Genome Project estimated that humans have around 30,000 protein-encoding genes, almost the same as a mouse yet, strangely, less than rice. When lengths of this DNA coil up very tightly around proteins known as histones, they form chromosomes. Each chromosome consists of two identical lengths of coiled DNA called chromatids, held together by a centromere, which gives it the appearance of two sausages pulled together by a string. The position of the centromere gives the chromosome its unique shape and is a useful marker for describing the location of specific genes. For example, geneticists might refer to the 'long arm' of the gene, which is located below the centromere, or the 'short arm' above the centromere. Humans, being what is called a diploid species, have 46 chromosomes arranged in 23 pairs – 23 from each parent. Of these, 22 have the same structure in males and females and are called autosomes. The twenty-third pair are the X (female) and Y (male) chromosomes, and define a person's sex – females have two X chromosomes and males an X and a Y.

The human genome is 6 billion base letters long, effectively making it an assembly of millions of combinations of A, C, G and T. As our cells inevitably divide or reproduce, they must take the instruction manual or genome with it, and thus our genome must be capable of reproducing itself in an infinite manner, through a process known as replication. Sometimes during replication, a base letter (for our purposes interchangeable with nucleotide) or group of base letters might be duplicated, deleted or damaged, causing a mutation in the code that may result in or contribute to a disease state.

Our genome contains the instruction manual or pattern book that determines our traits, but a number of other processes must take place to produce the physical manifestation of the given instruction. First, the information contained in the gene must be transcribed in the nucleus by a single-stranded ribonucleic acid (RNA) molecule, which carries the information away from the pattern book in the DNA, via messenger RNA, into the cytoplasm (body) of the cell, where the instructions will be converted into a unique sequence of amino acids via transfer RNA. Once the chain of amino acids has been correctly assembled and 'folded', it becomes a protein. Thus every protein that contributes to our traits originated from a message sent directly from our genome.

Our internally coded, inherited information is known as our genotype, while the outward expression or observable structure of this information is known as our phenotype. Our phenotype is genetic information made real, tangible and measurable. It includes our molecules, macromolecules, cells, tissues, organs, structures, metabolism and behaviours, and is unique to us. Our phenotype is also intimately linked to our environment. Although exactly how this interplay works is still largely unknown, many clues have emerged in recent years.

Genetics and disease

Genes play an important role in human diseases, which can be broadly sorted into two distinct categories. The first are monogenic or Mendelian inheritance diseases, which result from a single error or mutation in a single gene in our DNA and are classed as either dominant, recessive or X-linked. Dominant diseases involve damage to only one gene copy, while recessive diseases involve damage to both copies and X-linked diseases involve damage to a gene on the X chromosome, which are expressed only in males because they are not masked by a second X chromosome. Monogenic diseases include Tay-Sachs, sickle cell anaemia and cystic fibrosis, and are among scores of health conditions that run in families and can be detected by blood testing at birth.

Diseases in the second category are referred to as polygenic, multifactorial or non-Mendelian. These involve a sophisticated and often poorly understood interplay between our unique genetic variations and our specific environment. The 'big killers', such as heart disease, cancers, metabolic syndrome diseases and auto-immune diseases, fall into this category, as do the 'big disablers' of arthritis, obesity, asthma, depression, some intellectual disabil-ities and bowel diseases to name but a few. These diseases can also run in families, but the environmental components such as diet, lifestyle, stress, environmental toxins, viruses and radiation play a dominant role in determining whether or not an individual will succumb to the disease. In theory, these diseases have a strong element of preventability.

One of the most famous monogenic or inherited 'disease' genes is the HTT or 'huntingtin' gene, which is located on the short arm of chromosome 4, and provides instructions for making a protein called huntingtin. We all have an HTT gene that codes for huntingtin, and while the exact function of the protein is unknown, it's presumed to play a role in brain cells. In a non-affected person, one end of the HTT gene has a base combination of cytosine, adenine and guanine or CAG repeated ten to 35 times. When a mutation occurs, the repetition of this sequence will increase to between 36 and 120 CAG times. Those with 40 or more repeats generally go on to develop the condition known as Huntington disease. As the gene mutation is passed from one generation to the next, the number of faulty repeats increases, which may result in earlier onset of the condition in members of the subsequent generation – a phenomenon known as genetic anticipation.

Genes are grouped into 'families' that determine the types of proteins they will build. For example, the 54 functional KRT genes located on chromosomes 12 and 17 code for proteins called keratins, which form hair, skin, nails and the linings of internal organs. KRT genes are also involved in controlling cell size, growth and division, wound healing and internal cell movement. A variation in this gene could affect the expression of keratins, making hair or nails weaker.

The COLEC gene family on chromosome 10 provides instructions for making proteins called collectins, which are involved in the body's immune response to pathogens such as viruses, bacteria and yeasts. Collectin proteins feature a lectin region that recognises and binds to the carbohydrate structure on the surface of pathogens, and a collagen region that helps break down the pathogens and bind them together, preventing them from infecting more cells. Mutations or variations in the gene can contribute to autoimmune disorders or extreme susceptibility to repeat infections.

The effects of gene variations

One of the COLEC gene family members is the mannose-binding lectin gene (MBL2), which binds to mannose and N-acetylglucosamine sugars typically featured in large numbers on the surface of bacteria, fungi, viruses and protozoa. If this gene is defective, it prevents the body from producing sufficient MBL in the liver and secreting it into the bloodstream, rendering the immune system less effective at fighting and clearing pathogens.

MBL deficiency has been reported in numerous different populations, where 30 per cent of the population have less than 500 nanograms per millilitre of MBL when human levels may be as high as 10,000 nanograms per millilitre. This makes these people very susceptible to viruses that have N-acetylglucosamine sugars on their surface, such as Ebola, influenza, Marburg virus, SARS; and bacteria such as *Staphylococcus aureus*. MBL deficiency is associated with numerous health conditions, including autoimmune diseases such as IgA nephropathy, lupus, rheumatoid arthritis, respiratory diseases and atherosis, so the question of which genetic and environmental factors contribute to this apparently widespread problem of susceptibility to pathogens is an important one.

While the variation in the MBL2 gene can be found in scores of people, researchers know that not everyone with the variation will have insufficient MBL and not everyone with insufficient MBL will be prone to ongoing infections. Scientists believe that other genetic and environmental factors are involved in developing MBL deficiency and its many health consequences.

Epigenetics

The variations or mutations in genes such as MBL2 are often referred to as epigenetic. Epigenetics is the study of the changes that happen inside cells that determine which genes will be turned on and which genes will be turned off. When a gene is turned on, it becomes active and is able to do its job: being expressed to produce a protein. When a gene is turned off, it's still available but is no longer active and performing its function. It's important to note that genes are not just responsible for performing a function but are part of a *process* that involves other functioning or malfunctioning genes. Scientists studying epigenetics are interested in factors that can alter gene expression, namely DNA methylation, histone modification and chromatin remodelling.

WHAT IS METHYLATION?

A methyl group is a carbon atom with three hydrogens attached and has the capacity to bind to numerous molecules within the body. Molecules with a methyl group that can pass it on to another molecule are called methyl donors, and the process is called methylation.

In DNA methylation, methyl groups are added to DNA, which modifies its function. Appropriate methylation is critical for numerous cell processes and gene expression, but aberrant methylation patterns (too much or too little) are almost always found in cancerous tissues in the colon, stomach, cervix, breast and prostate and thyroid glands.

Variations such as MBL2 are known as single-nucleotide polymorphisms (SNPs) and number between 10 million and possibly 30 million, in the human genome. These epigenetic markers represent an alteration to a single nucleotide in the DNA sequence; for example, an 'SNP may replace the nucleotide cytosine (C) with the nucleotide thymine (T) in a certain stretch of DNA' and this may alter the functional aspect of the gene. While we all possess SNPs that are known to confer a multitude of disease risks, researchers have noted that genetic architecture is large, multilayered and hugely complex. This means perhaps that relying on genetics to predict disease may be akin to trying to 'predict the unpredictable'.

The exposome

Perhaps a more realistic goal may involve identifying not just the genetic straw or rather collection of straws that will ultimately break the camel's back, but the modifiable environmental determinants that might prevent the camel's back from breaking at all. The 'exposome' has been proposed as a potential unifying framework that encompasses the sum of all human environmental exposures, from the point of conception onwards, that may impact or influence the genome. The exposome brings together environmental factors such diet, pollutants and pharmaceuticals, and lifestyle factors such as chronic stress, which may ultimately have an impact on our genetic expression. Altering an exposome is infinitely easier than changing a genome, and it may prove to be an effective way to prevent and treat disease or substantially ameliorate symptoms where the cause of the illness is identified.

While the genetic architectures of Westernised populations are clearly struggling to function in the face of complex exposomes made up of numerous environmental insults, Weston Price's study subjects were not. These people were primarily dealing with the terrible impact of sugar and refined wheat on their ancient and previously robust genomic architectures, and yet the consequence of this dietary insult was obvious for all to see. With the limited scientific insight available during his era, Price attributed this situation to the displacing effects of sugar and refined wheat; in other words, he proposed that indigenous populations, which typically consumed nutrient-dense foods drawn from their natural surroundings, developed a preference for nutrient-devoid 'white man's food' when it became available, in effect 'displacing' the traditional foods that had long protected their health.

Nutrigenetics and nutrigenomics

The HGP and the subsequent identification of SNPs associated with disease have opened up fascinating new areas of science such as nutrigenetics and nutrigenomics. Nutrigenetics refers to the role of variations in the DNA sequence in response to dietary chemicals (nutrients). Specifically, nutrigenetics looks at mutations or variations in genes involved in both the metabolism of nutrients and in the metabolic pathways dependent on micronutrients (such as vitamins), as well as the epigenetic process of genes being turned on or off in response to diet or other aspects of the exposome. For example, abnormal DNA or histone methylation resulting from deficiency or poor regulation of the methyl donors folate, vitamins B2, B6, B12, zinc, selenium, choline and methionine is thought to contribute to many health disorders.

Nutrigenomics refers to the effect of dietary chemicals (nutrients) on gene expression. This includes genome instability, which can result from damage to the DNA at the chromosomal and molecular level, such as breaks in the DNA strand or telomere damage; epigenetic alterations such as DNA methylation; RNA and microRNA expression; protein expression; and metabolite (the products of metabolism) alteration.

Both nutrigenetics and nutrigenomics are predicated upon the understanding that throughout the evolution of mankind, diet would likely have affected gene expression. This may have resulted in phenotypes that were better adapted to various environmental challenges and that enabled better utilisation of food resources, ultimately resulting in stronger and more robust humans. In addition, individual differences may exist in terms of responsiveness to repeated, ongoing exposure to given nutrients. One example is the discovery by geneticist Rasmus Nielsen at the University of California that Inuit people have unique variations in the genes associated with enzymes that help regulate different fats in the body. The Inuit diet has been rich in omega-3 fat for 20,000 years, so the gene may have altered its expression or adapted to maintain blood levels of fatty acids in a safe balance. Only 2 per cent of Europeans share this gene variant.

According to researchers at the cutting edge of nutrigenetics and nutrigenomics, several tenets underpin three fundamental hypotheses:

1. Nutrition may impact health directly, by affecting gene expression in essential metabolic pathways, or indirectly, by influencing genetic mutation at the nucleotide or chromosome level, which in turn may impact gene dosage (number of copies), and gene expression.

2. The health benefits associated with nutrients and nutrient combinations rely on genetic variants that affect the way the cells take up nutrients and metabolise them, or interact with individual molecules involved in metabolic processes.

3. Dietary intervention based upon an individual's inherited and acquired genetic characteristics, nutritional requirements, nutritional status, life stage, dietary preferences and health status can be individualised with a view to preventing, ameliorating or curing chronic disease.

The notion that diet can impact genetic expression has long been understood. This is the case for galactosemia, a condition in which a recessive defect in the gene that codes for an enzyme called galactose-1-phosphate uridyltransferase (GALT) results in accumulation of the sugar galactose in the blood, leading to health problems such as mental retardation. The condition is screened for at birth and managed with a low-lactose diet (as most dietary galactose comes from lactose, which is a double sugar comprised one glucose molecule bound to one galactose molecule). A recessive defect in the gene that codes for the enzyme phenylalanine hydroxylase results in phenylketonuria, which manifests as an accumulation of the amino acid phenylalanine in the blood, potentially causing neurological damage. The condition is managed with a low-phenylalanine diet (largely a low-protein diet).

FOOD AND GENETIC EXPRESSION:
THE CASE OF HARRY'S HAIR

Through an accidental discovery with our family dog, Harry, I was able to observe an interesting case of how an environmental input, namely diet, can overcome genetic programming.

Harry, a chocolate spoodle, inherited a white chest patch from his father and, as we found out six months after purchasing him, a grey streak of fur down his back from his mother. Resigned to having a prematurely greying puppy, we figured there wasn't much we could do about it – it was an obvious case of genetic anticipation and we should accept his fate!

Our dog's 'high-quality' diet at that point consisted of raw meat, bones, carrots and broccoli, dried or cooked locally produced human-grade chicken, fresh boneless fish and a high-quality

---

Australian-made gluten-free dog crunch. Harry only drank water, but if he could manage occasionally to score himself a bit of thick cream from the rim of the milk container, he was really in heaven.

Without thinking too much about it, I started purchasing an air-dried beef-liver crunch made locally using human-grade beef. I viewed the crunch as little more than a snack to add variety to our dog's diet. When I gave Harry the beef-liver crunch, however, he ate significant amounts of it, almost as though he was desperate for something it contained. After a while, I would just leave a few pieces out for him and he would ignore them for days before finally eating them and then looking around for more. To me this indicated that he instinctively knew he had a requirement for the nutrients contained in the beef liver, but also knew when he had received enough or needed a top-up.

I still didn't think anything of it until Hairy Harry went for a much-needed grooming session in which his fur was shorn to a length of just a few millimetres. We were puzzled when the newly shaved Harry was returned to us with a beautiful glossy, velvety, deep-chocolate coat – without any grey hair.

I didn't make the connection between the disappearance of the 'inherited' grey hair and the beef liver until I was unable to purchase from the usual supplier and had to buy a standard pet-shop brand. After a few weeks eating the pet-shop brand, Harry's grey hair started to grow through again. When I finally caught up with my usual supplier of beef liver, I explained the strange turn of events to her. She was not at all surprised, telling me that her beef liver had intentionally been air-dried in order to retain maximum density of nutrients. In Harry's case this was B-group vitamins; vitamin K; zinc, iron, the amino acids taurine, leucine and cysteine; and the methyl donors for DNA repair B-vitamins choline and folate, and amino acid methionine. I purchased a large supply from her, and from that point on Harry has only been given this particular beef.

As I sit here typing, Harry has just returned from the groomers to shed seven months of winter fleece, and his new velvety growth is a deep, rich and glossy chocolate colour – still without grey hair. With a nutrient-dense diet, it would appear that Harry has been able to defy his genetic programming. What if we could all be like Harry?

A nutrient-dense diet as treatment

With this modern-day understanding of how diet can influence our gene expression and hence our propensity to manifest disease, it becomes easier to understand the claims by Weston Price and the doctors attending the indigenous populations that nutrient-dense indigenous diets were capable of restoring health to these individuals. But what about modern-day populations? Can nutrient-dense diets break the cycle of chronic disease that currently threatens to crash our health system?

In 2015, a group of nutrition specialists from both academia and industry met at the University Medical Center in the Netherlands to discuss the nutritional situation of the general public and its connection to the rise in non-communicable or chronic disease. The group noted that even in affluent countries, more than 75 per cent of adults did not meet the recommended intakes for a considerable number of vitamins, while more than half of German infants and children under the age of five were also below the recommended intake of vitamins D, E, C and folate. An analysis of Swiss children aged nine to nineteen found that between 10 per cent and almost 70 per cent of children failed to meet the recommendations for vitamins A, B6, B12, C, E, thiamine (B1), riboflavin (B2), folate (B12), niacin (B3) and pantothenic acid (B5). Given the crucial role of several of these vitamins in DNA methylation, this is quite a worrying observation. In addition, the group noted that the children were only tested for protein-related vitamin deficiencies, and that the rates of malnutrition would be manifestly higher if additional micronutrient or mineral deficiencies were taken into consideration.

Like Weston Price, the nutrition specialists noted that increased consumption of sugary drinks, while not just linked to obesity and insulin resistance, served to deprive individuals of vitamins and minerals thanks to their ability to displace nutrient density with energy density. The group concluded that a shift from energy density to nutrient density might help citizens lower their risk of developing non-communicable diseases and enjoy a longer life of greater quality. The group recognises that nutrient density may be the best way to break the intergenerational cycle of malnutrition and obesity, and cites programs such the introduction in Canada of affordable, nutrient-dense, tasty and filling lunch bags for schools as one way of decreasing children's desire to snack on junk food.

The low nutrient intake among such large numbers of the population is interesting in terms of the high levels of depression being reported around the world. In a 2015 review paper titled 'What if nutrients could treat mental illness?', researchers noted a decade's worth of studies showing an improvement in symptoms – including irritability, depression and anxiety – upon supplementation with vitamin and mineral preparations. This reflects other research demonstrating that diets high in vegetables and fruits are associated with fewer symptoms of anxiety and depression, while diets high in processed foods and low in vegetables and fruits are related to an increased in symptoms.

The rise in rates of depression around the world has led to a dramatic increase in the prescription of medications, many of which are now being revealed as potentially problematic. A 2015 systematic review of the carcinogenetic properties of psychotropic drugs in animal studies found that 90 per cent of new-generation antipsychotics and anticonvulsants, 63.6 per cent of antidepressants and 70 per cent of benzodiazepines and other sedative-hypnotics showed evidence of carcinogenicity. In light of these findings, perhaps nutrient density should become one of the first therapeutic options made available to people, particularly pregnant women, children and young people and those with a family history of cancer.

The human microbiome

While the sequencing of the human genome was a landmark achievement in science, and has led to additional breakthroughs in how foods interact with genes to influence phenotype and disease susceptibility, human genomics in and of itself is only a partial tool for understanding human biology. Unravelling the symbiotic relationship between humans and the microbes living in and on them presents yet another great frontier in understanding human health.

In 2008, the US NIH launched the Human Microbiome Project (HMP) with the goal of identifying and characterising the microbial communities that reside in the human gut, mouth, nasal passages, lungs and vagina, as well as on the skin. One of the most startling data points to emerge from this study was the understanding that we are more microbial than we are human: the total microbial cell count outnumbers the human cell count by ten to one, while the genes associated with these microbes outnumber the human gene count by 100 to one. This realisation has given rise to the idea of the human body as a superorganism possessed of a 'distributed intelligence', in which individual life forms with limited information are able to work together to accomplish a goal beyond that of serving the individual, such as survival of the whole. The superorganism exemplifies the notion of collaboration and of putting the interests of the whole above self-interest. This in turn is reshaping how scientists understand human health and disease.

The HMP has enabled scientists to begin to elucidate the impact of genetics, prenatal timing and mode of birth, infant feeding patterns, antibiotic usage, smoking, cleanliness of living conditions and lifetime dietary patterns on the intestinal microbial communities that, as it turns out, may play a vital role in our health. By far, the largest microbial populations inhabit the gastrointestinal tract – in particular the colon.

Scientists know that the most dominant bacterial groups in the gut are the Bacteroidetes, Firmicutes and Actinobacteria. The gut bacteria are known to play an important role in facilitating the development and maturation of the immune system, protecting against pathogens, fermenting fibrous food components and harvesting nutrients. Aberrant alterations to the composition of gut bacteria is known as 'dysbiosis'. Reduced abundance and diversity of Firmicutes, for example, has been noted in individuals with Crohn's disease, while a reduced number of one species of Firmicutes, known as *Faecalibacterium prausnitzii*, has been associated with a higher risk of post-operative recurrence of Crohn's symptoms.

The microbiome and infant health

The story of our microbial community begins while we are still in the womb. During this time, our mother's gut and vaginal bacterial community is remodelled, possibly in response to hormonal changes. This vast community (sometimes referred to as our 'old friend') is seeded at birth, evolving for better or worse throughout our lifetime. It's passed to us as a type of living genetic inheritance from our mothers as we move through the birth canal, make contact with her skin and receive our first nourishment through breastmilk. We are life partners with our microbiome and yet, if not for the recent upsurge of research in this area, we would scarcely have been aware of its presence.

While it has long been supposed that the earliest transmission of the microbial community from mother to infant occurs during the passage down the birth canal, augmented by microbes from the mother's skin and breastmilk, recent research would indicate that some bacteria can bypass the placental and amniotic barriers and gain entry to the developing foetus, possibly via the mouth and the bloodstream. Researchers fed pregnant mice milk that had been laced with genetically labelled *Enterococcus faecium* bacteria before delivering their offspring via caesarean section one day before a natural delivery was to occur. Not only did the first bowel movement of the baby mice contain bacteria, but some of those bacteria carried the genetic label and could therefore only have reached the babies from the mouth or gut of their mother.

During vaginal delivery, the infant is exposed to the microbes in the mother's vagina and gut. Recent research conducted at the Yakult Honsha European Research Center in Belgium, and thus funded by the manufacturer of Yakult probiotic drinks, isolated 2500 strains of bifidobacteria from the faeces of mothers before delivery, and from their baby's meconium and faeces at days three, seven, 30 and 90 after birth. Eighty-two of the mother–baby pairs were born by vaginal delivery and 29 by caesarean delivery. The researchers demonstrated that certain strains of the beneficial bifidobacteria were both predominant and stable in the mother's gut before the transmission, and that colonisation of specific strains took place during and after birth. No such transmission was observed in the caesarean delivery group. This is worrying given the modern frequency of caesarean births and that bifidobacteria (in addition to lactobacilli) provide several essential services to the newborn: preventing the colonisation of the baby's gut by pathogenic bacteria; and helping build and maintain the newly developing immune system. They provide essential vitamins to the newborn, and increase the tight junctions between the gut and blood vessels, which is potentially vital to the cognitive health of the infant.

This essential colonisation of the newborn by bifidobacterium strains has a 200-million-year history, and so it remains to be seen how the huge numbers of caesarean births that have occurred over the last twenty years will ultimately play out in the health of these children as they live their lives. In one study of Iranian babies, the differences in the microbial communities of those delivered via vaginal versus caesarean births was still present at the age of seven. Researchers already know that caesarean babies are at increased risk of asthma, allergic reactions, food sensitivities, type 1 diabetes, eczema, obesity and necrotising enterocolitis (potentially fatal tissue death in parts of the intestines) as a result of reduced bacterial richness and diversity, reduced colonisation of beneficial bacteria and increased colonisation of potential pathogens at birth. Given that the gut is a primary entry point for invading pathogens, a robust microbiome structure from birth would seem vital to long-term health.

Yet another startling finding regarding the importance of the bifidobacteria colonisation process is that some of the sugars in the mother's breastmilk are indigestible by the infant, but instead are there to feed the bacteria that in turn help the baby develop properly. In addition, the sugars in breastmilk prevent pathogens from attaching to healthy cells. Breastmilk itself has been found to contain up to 600 species of bacteria, including bifidobacteria and lactobacilli, along with nutrients and maternal antibodies to protect against disease. None of these are present in formula milk. Research from Iran has shown that younger women and women from rural areas tend to have more lactobacilli in their breastmilk, indicating that age and diet (that is, greater consumption of traditional fermented foods among rural populations) is likely to assist the development of the baby's immune system. The Yakult researchers noted that it might be very important for women to build and maintain a very healthy microbiota during pregnancy in preparation for the transmission of a healthy microbiome to their new arrivals.

While vaginally delivered babies acquire the microbial community that most reflects their passage into the world, caesarean-born babies acquire a microbial community most like the maternal skin, such as *Staphylococcus*, *Corynebacterium* and *Propionibacterium*. This is an important observation, because a three-year study of 164 babies who had a first-degree relative with coeliac disease looked at whether the babies had the gene variations, called HLA-DQ, that put them at risk of developing the disease. The study also considered diet and faecal bacteria at day seven, one month and four months old. Early results demonstrated that regardless of breast- or formula feeding, these genetically susceptible babies had lower numbers of *Bifidobacterium* and higher numbers of *Staphylococcus*, indicating that the host's HLA-DQ genes appeared to favour colonisation by the latter. In addition, a study into the gut microbiome of sudden infant death syndrome (SIDS) babies found that they were more likely to be colonised by *Staphylococcus aureus*, *Clostridium difficile* and *Clostridium perfringens*, all of which can cause illness.

Over the first three years after birth, the child will develop its predominant microbial structure as it moves to consuming solid foods of different varieties. Research has suggested that long-term diet is the primary driver of the microbial communities in the gut, and that changes in diet are the easiest way to modify these communities in most people. Given the lack of research into how host genetics, diet and gut microbiota work together in promoting health, however, it's difficult to know which interventions are most effective and longest lasting.

The adult microbiome

The mature adult intestinal microbiome predominantly comprises bacteria from six or seven main groups, 80 per cent of which can be identified as members of the Bacteroidetes, Firmicutes or Actinobacteria. The Bacteroidetes and Firmicutes exist in a yin-and-yang-style ratio; the microbiota of obese research subjects have revealed greater numbers of Firmicutes and fewer Bacteroidetes, while the opposite ratio has been linked to weight loss. Faecal analysis of the microbiota of lupus patients revealed higher levels of Bacteroidetes and lower levels of Firmicutes, in a ratio similar to that found in people with Crohn's disease or type 2 diabetes.

Bacteroidetes are a very diverse group of 7000 different bacterial species. Gut Bacteroidetes generally manufacture short-chain fatty acids such as butyrate, acetate and propionate through fermentation of dietary fibres. Butyrate itself is understood to prevent and inhibit colorectal cancer and may exert positive effects on genetic metabolic diseases, insulin resistance, high blood cholesterol and stroke.

Firmicutes, also known as lactic acid bacteria, are particularly well suited to living on sugar, so the more sugars and processed carbohydrates we eat, the happier Firmicutes appear to be. In fact, the more we eat generally, the happier Firmicutes are, hence their links to obesity.

Because Weston Price's research subjects have now experienced the full effects of Westernisation, it's difficult to know what type of microbial communities existed in and on their bodies before the arrival of 'white man'. With very few truly untouched indigenous communities left in the world, the task of finding an unmodernised microbiome would seem an unlikely quest – if not for the eagle eye of a Venezuelan military helicopter. The High Orinoco area of the Amazonas Region of Venezuela comprises roughly 80,000 square kilometres of dense jungle, which provides sanctuary for 15,000 indigenous Yanomami people. Most of these live in riverside villages and are partially modernised. What the military helicopter spotted, however, was a group of 54 Yanomami 'research subjects' between the ages of four and 50 who, after more than 11,000 years of isolation, were still living the true hunter-gatherer existence in remote areas. They should perhaps have been left alone completely, but a research team went in and examined their lifestyle and microbiota.

The group had no domestication of animals, did not engage in agriculture and had no prior contact with humans apart from other remote Yanomami. The research team noted the group's Paleo-style diet of foraged wild bananas, seasonal fruits, plantain, palm hearts, cassava, birds, small mammals, crabs, frogs, small fish from local streams, peccaries (native pigs), monkeys and tapirs, and that they collected water from a stream located a short walk from the village. This Yanomami group had evidently flourished, despite excluding entire food groups, such as dairy, grains and legumes, from their diet. The visiting scientific group took bacterial samples from the inside forearm skin, oral mucosa and faeces of 34 of the 54 villagers.

The research team, which included Martin J. Blaser, director of the Human Microbiome Program at New York University and author of the book *Missing Microbes*, published a number of startling insights. Despite no known exposure to antibiotics (apart from one instance of a strange choice by the scientists, who were there to obtain samples of a rare and unique collection of intestinal microbes, to administer antibiotics known to harm the microbiota) the group had functional antibiotic-resistance genes, including those that confer resistance to synthetic antibiotics. The Yanomami faecal microbiota was characterised by high levels of Prevotella and low levels of Bacteroides, which was similar to the microbiota of the Guahibo Amerindians, Malawians and other African hunter-gatherers, and the exact opposite to that found in

US subjects. Even more fascinating is that the isolated Yanomami maintained a microbiome with the 'highest diversity of bacteria and genetic functions ever reported in a human group'.

Given their propensity to wander naked in their environment, their skin profile featured organic acids, amino acids, vitamins, methane and a diverse skin microbiota. This skin microbiota was in stark contrast to that of US subjects, which was more likely to have a low diversity and feature high numbers of *Staphylococcus*, *Corynebacterium*, *Neisseria* and *Propionibacterium*, no doubt due to clothing, antibacterial washes, soaps, chemicals and other features of our modern-day exposome.

Microbiota diversity and health

A growing body of research has suggested that a gut microbiota of low diversity may lead to negative health consequences. In addition, low bacterial diversity at birth may set the scene for a malfunctioning immune system down the track. So how does the average American microbiome, born and bred on the standard American diet filled with sugar, refined wheat and seed oils, compare with those of not just the Yanomami but also other indigenous peoples?

A group of researchers compared the faecal microbiomes of three geographically dispersed groups: healthy Amerindians from the Amazonas of Venezuela; residents of rural Malawian communities; and inhabitants of a US metropolitan area. The results revealed little difference between the groups up to the age of three years, but from then on, the microbial profile of the US subjects became much less diverse with fewer species. Fewer species means a lower number of genes associated with the individual bacterial species, and research has revealed a link between low bacterial gene count and increased risk of obesity, insulin resistance, high levels of fat in the blood and inflammation. In addition, researchers have noted that people with low bacterial gene counts fail to respond satisfactorily to nutritional intervention with a low-fat, high-protein, complex-carbohydrate, fibrous plant-based diet. Diseases associated with low species and gene counts within the intestinal microbiota include type 1 and type 2 diabetes, coeliac disease, autism, cystic fibrosis, allergies and *Clostridium difficile* infection.

Could this be why so many people who fail to lose weight suddenly lose weight effortlessly when they radically change their diet? Could this be why people recover from some symptoms of disease and autoimmunity when they do the same? Could one of the secrets to Paleo diets (devoid of sugar, grains and processed foods, and rich in nutritious plant life, fermented foods, nuts and grass-fed meats) be that they enable the microbiome to recover diversity, function and gene count sufficiently to help people regain their health? Should we be looking to the wisdom of the untouched Yanomami for inspiration to guide us out of this chronic-disease mess?

From René Dubos's early attempts to warn us about the risks inherent in straying too far from our relationship with our natural world, to the discovery of the 'shop manual of medicine' and its subsequent insights into the teeming microbial world within us all, it would seem that once again the evidence points to the importance of what we choose to put into our mouths, and how its contents affect not just our genes, but the genes of our enduring microbial community. We already know that many doctors don't deal in diets, and in the coming chapters you will learn that industry-sponsored dietitians specifically don't deal in Yanomami diets. On the surface it may appear that we are collectively stuck between a rock and a hard place, but as Chapter 9 outlines, ordinary people are on the move, finding new health authorities and doing it for themselves.

What can our genome reveal?

When I finished writing the bulk of this chapter, I became very curious about what my own genome might reveal, and so I decided to take a genomic wellness test and find out. Friends asked me if I was crazy. Why would I want to find out about even more health conditions I might have, given the problems I have already had to deal with? Wouldn't it scare me? Wouldn't I rather just not know?

Having spent hundreds of hours wading around in the latest books and scientific literature on genetics during the course of writing this chapter, I already knew that no matter what I found, it would be unlikely to scare me. Numerous experts in the field have noted that our genetic architecture is large and complex – simply having a particular gene would not be a guarantee of anything. In addition, given that our environment can have an impact on our genetic expression, I figured that knowing what was locked inside my own black box of genetic data could in fact be empowering. Maybe I could fiddle with my environment and make my genes work for me.

The test itself involved sending off a test tube with a glob of saliva in the bottom to a laboratory and scheduling an appointment with a health professional trained in interpreting the results. It took about one month to receive the results, which covered areas such as fat metabolism, vitamin metabolism, food responses, methylation, liver detoxification mechanisms, weight management, response to exercise and the risk of developing cardiovascular disease and type 2 diabetes.

Folate metabolism

When my results came back, the first thing I was interested in was finding out whether I had the dreaded mutation in the gene for the enzyme methylenetetrahydrofolate reductase (MTHFR) on chromosome 1, which affects how much active folate is available to my cells. Because folate (vitamin B9) is required for so many cell processes, problems with the MTHFR gene can lead us down the road to chronic disease. There is a lot of information on the web on MTHFR (and a little on page 257), mainly because the mutation is believed to be involved in many health conditions and it's one mutation in which supplementation with B vitamins may assist. In the event, I turned out to be officially off the hook for this one.

Type 2 diabetes

The second thing I was interested in finding out was whether I was at risk of type 2 diabetes. While type 2 diabetes is exceedingly rare in my family, the steep rise in the condition throughout the West would indicate that environmental factors such as diet are now playing a role. I wanted to see if I could gain any further insights into how to avoid symptoms of the precursor condition metabolic syndrome. I also wanted to know what type of diet would best suit me, as historically I have always weighed less and had more energy on a higher protein, moderate-fat and lower carbohydrate diet, while I tend to bloat and gain weight quickly if I eat carbohydrates in the form of bread, pasta, rice and potatoes, even if the grain used is gluten-free.

Sure enough, despite having only one distant family member who developed type 2 diabetes, I had a stack of genes indicating I was very much at risk of winding up with metabolic syndrome and impaired insulin response, which could in turn lead me to develop type 2 diabetes. This is definitely not a situation I would be happy with! While a super-low-carb or ketogenic diet would not be necessary for me, the genome test certainly confirmed that the high-carbohydrate diet recommended by the government of six slices of bread and five serves of vegetables and legumes a day would certainly cause problems for me in the long run. One diet does not fit all, and it would appear that genetic testing may finally put an end to an ineffective nationally standardised prescribed diet and firmly place the personalisation of diet on the map.

Coffee, sugar and salt

I do love my daily coffee, but research into genetics has indicated that people who metabolise caffeine too slowly and yet continue to drink it are at increased risk of organ damage – something I definitely do not want any more of! As it turned out, I am a fast metaboliser of caffeine, so I was off the hook again.

I wouldn't describe myself as a sugar addict, which makes sense because as it turns out I don't have the 'sugar gene' SNP, which predisposes people to becoming hooked on sugar. Once when I attended a night AFL game, I needed to take my transplant tablets but didn't have any water. I either had to brave the food outlet crowd to buy water, or drink some lemonade from a bottle belonging to a friend. I chose the latter option and absent-mindedly took a large gulp to wash down the pills. As soon as the sugar hit my mouth the reaction was violent – the drink and the pills spurted out all over the ground. The sugary taste was unbelievable. 'How do you drink this stuff?' I sputtered to my shocked friend.

Because I take my own blood pressure on a regular basis, I had noticed that when I consume salty processed foods such as hot chips, my blood pressure goes up and takes quite a while to normalise again. I often wondered why this might be the case, but it turns out that I have SNPs for salt sensitivity and hypertension. The only way for me to truly avoid health problems associated with added sodium is to avoid processed food altogether. It's worth noting that I do add mineralised salt to my cooking and this has no negative effect on my blood pressure.

Stress response

One of the most exasperating aspects of my life as a chronic-disease patient is that I have what is known as 'white coat hypertension', which means that every time I clap eyes on a doctor, my blood pressure goes ridiculously high – as in 180/120! I always imagine that they are about announce some terrible news I don't want to hear, and it puts my system into high alert. Once I am in the comfort of my own home, however, it hums along at a very reliable 115/75. My efforts to convince doctors that this is the case are usually met with raised eyebrows. But who would have thought a gene test would ultimately vindicate my claims? As it turns out, I have SNPs involved in my stress response genes that facilitate the 'white coat hypertension' phenomenon. In reality, it might be better described as a fight or flight response – and in my case it's definitely flight.

Vitamins and minerals

Experts are now telling us that a few minutes a day in the sun is sufficient to get enough vitamin D. Once again, this is a one-size-fits-all recommendation that might be beneficial to some while very hazardous to others. My gene SNPs, however, demonstrated that I am at an increased risk of vitamin D deficiency (a problem given it's involved in the expression of 900 genes) and so require a daily dose of sunshine along with dietary sources such as eggs, fish, mushrooms or supplements. What the 'two minutes a day' experts also forget is that a daily dose of sunshine makes us feel better. There is nothing greater for the body, the mind and our stress levels than taking a nice walk in the sun and breathing in fresh air. I always feel much happier after a daily dose of sunshine, and now I know why – I have the SNPs that make me more likely to be affected by seasonal affective disorder or SADS, which is also known as the 'I hate winter' syndrome. And I do – so no surprises there. If I could follow the sun, I would!

While some people argue that vitamin supplementation is unnecessary (and that everything should come from the diet) and others contend that supplements are great, I would suggest that every argument involves three people – those at either end and the person in the middle. On the subject of supplementation, I sit firmly in the middle and this is why. Not only do our individual genes play a role in determining adequate vitamin and mineral levels, but so does our individual environment, and certain factors can increase demand. For example, ACE inhibitors and corticosteroid medications such as those used to treat high blood pressure, some heart conditions and autoimmune diseases (and transplants!) increase urinary zinc secretion. This means that not only is less zinc available for repairing tissue damaged by autoimmunity itself, but cell membranes are also weakened and are less effective in defending against the pathogens often involved in chronic infections and autoimmunity. Zinc deficiency is considered to be at pandemic proportions in both developed and developing countries. Soils in most parts of the world are depleted of the mineral, and bioavailability in common foods ranges from 10 to 30 per cent. Common foods such as wheat contain phytates, which interfere with zinc uptake, while excess sugar consumption can inhibit zinc absorption. In addition, people can have hereditary forms of zinc deficiency without knowing it. In such a case, diet will never be enough to maintain the stores and supplementation will be necessary. My own blood tests show that I have immense trouble maintaining zinc stores through diet alone, and that I need regular supplements to maintain correct levels.

Another vitamin I need to supplement is vitamin C, as I have several SNPs that indicate an increased risk of deficiency if I fail to maintain solid dietary levels. Low levels of vitamin C can lead to prolonged infections, which would be dangerous for somebody in my position. In addition, adequate vitamin C levels decrease the risk of several cancers, including bladder, breast, ovarian, cervical, colorectal, lung and head, neck and oesophageal cancers. My secret trick to upping my vitamin c is to pick up a tub of organic blueberries from the farmers' market each week and simply crunch my way through a large handful while they are still frozen. I end up with blue lips – but it's a small price to pay and it washes off.

While eggs and almonds are a regular part of my diet, the fact that I carry an SNP linked to lower blood levels of the antioxidant alpha-Tocopherol (a form of vitamin E) means that I should maintain these foods as part of my diet. If I don't, I would probably need to take a good-quality vitamin E supplement.

The genome testing sequence does not provide information on SNPs that are involved in minerals, but I think such a test would be beneficial for many people. With micronutrient deficiencies already rife in many societies, knowing if you carry SNPs associated with a need for higher intakes would add another layer of personalisation that could prevent, ameliorate or even cure some illnesses. Perhaps in the future a complete nutritional gene test will be available for consumers.

Physical activity

Genome testing can also provide clues regarding the best type of exercise for your unique profile. My results finally shed light on some of the mysteries surrounding why my body would respond to exercise differently and why exercise on its own has little bearing on my weight but a big impact on my muscles.

In terms of sport, I have never enjoyed activities that require a long, hard slog. The mere thought of marathon running would make me nauseous. While many people love nothing more than to run each day for fitness, I prefer sprinting and activities that involve short bursts with small breaks in between – such as tennis or badminton.

As it turns out I have a number of SNPs associated with type II or fast-twitch muscle fibres, which make me better matched to sprint performance. This means exercise such as tennis, basketball, light weights, yoga or short-distance running is more beneficial for me. High-intensity interval training (HIIT) would probably be another fitness option for my gene profile. HIIT involves doing a set number of exercises, each of which is performed in rapid succession for 20–30 seconds, and resting between each set for ten seconds. Sport scientists say that this efficient method of exercise will improve insulin sensitivity, decrease body fat, and boost endurance and muscular fitness. The high-intensity nature of the exercise means that you should probably talk to your doctor before trying it if you haven't exercised for a long time or have a health problem.

When I was younger (much younger!) I used to swim laps for 1.5 kilometres before I went to work. This type of marathon was fine and good stress reliever, but my weight never changed and I very quickly built up huge shoulder muscles, which really wasn't the look I was going for at the time. I gave the swimming up and my shoulders returned to their normal size. My gene test revealed that I should never have bothered with slow, continuous lap swimming and would have been much better off swimming shorter distances at a faster speed, which would also have been more practical, as it would have saved me time.

A tailored-health future

While my gene test provided personalised health information in addition to what I have discussed here, I hope this overview has demonstrated how knowing a bit more about how our body is programmed can help us understand why it behaves the way it does under certain conditions. If I had known years ago that I had the SNP for 'white coat hypertension', it would have saved me a lot of stress as a patient dealing with different doctors with different belief systems about my health issues. Knowing that I may have trouble maintaining correct levels of nutrients such as zinc, vitamin C or vitamin D means I can make the extra effort to keep myself topped up via my diet or supplementation. Knowing which diet and which exercise plan to follow for generating the best weight and metabolic profile means that I no longer have to experiment or take notice of fad diets or standardised dietary guidelines that would actually be harmful to my genetic profile. This type of genetic testing shows that one size will never fit all and personalisation is here to stay.

5

Can seed oils make us sick?

In recent times the reputations of sugar, wheat and 'bad' fats – seed oils – have taken a public battering and these foods are now shunned as a matter of course by many in the wellness community. It seems ironic that the three main foods given to Weston Price's indigenous cohort by colonial traders are today the three foods increasingly on the hit list of health-conscious consumers.

As previously discussed, Price's research subjects were aware of the damage being inflicted upon their health by the 'store' staples of sugar, wheat and seed oils. That several diseases or indicators of diminished health became common to all fourteen groups despite their different physical locations, genetic variations and previous indigenous diets is quite remarkable. For this reason, each of these foods deserves closer inspection.

When I first started writing this book, I was mostly interested in the sugar and refined-wheat part of the equation, given that Price's subjects would likely have consumed larger amounts of these than they would have seed oils. What I didn't realise, however, is that it doesn't take a lot of seed oil to negatively impact the human body.

The more I looked at the history, politics and science of fats, the more I came to realise that the long legacy of misinformation concerning them has undoubtedly contributed to a now-global public-health disaster of unprecedented proportions. The small amount of seed oil given to Price's indigenous groups could conceivably have been involved in their reports of arthritis, bone problems, maternal health problems and increased behavioural and psychiatric problems, but the scale on which seed oils are consumed as part of the Western diet far surpasses those amounts.

Today's rapidly increasing scale of global consumption, combined with the known negative health effects of seed oils – or more specifically the omega-6 or linoleic acid contained in soybean, cottonseed, corn, sunflower and safflower oils – on so many systems within the human body makes its ubiquitous but little-known presence in the food supply very alarming. The more I learned about seed oils, why we consume so much of them and their role in chronic disease, the more I realised that it may just be one of the biggest stories never told.

WHAT ARE OMEGA-3 AND OMEGA-6 FATTY ACIDS?

The basic components of fats, sometimes referred to as lipids, are molecules called fatty acids. These are more or less straight chains of carbon atoms with hydrogen atoms attached along most of their length and what is called a carboxyl group at one end. This carboxyl group is what characterises these hydrocarbon chains as acids.

In *saturated* fatty acids, all the carbon-to-carbon bonds along the length of the fatty acid are single bonds and have the maximum number of hydrogen atoms attached – in other words, they are 'saturated' with hydrogen.

In *unsaturated* fatty acids, there is at least one double carbon bond (a stronger bond, with two fewer attached hydrogen atoms) along the length. One of these double carbon bonds makes the fatty acid *monounsaturated*; more than one and they are *polyunsaturated*.

Where one of the double bonds in a polyunsaturated fatty acid occurs at position 3 along its length (between the third and fourth carbon atoms from the non-carboxyl end), it's called an omega-3 fatty acid. When it occurs at position 6 along its length (between the sixth and seventh carbon atoms from the non-carboxyl end), it's called an omega-6 fatty acid. The most common omega-6 fatty acid found in seed oils and other plant foods is linoleic acid.

The 'bad' fats debate

The seed oils that the trade winds delivered to Price's indigenous research subjects was likely in the form of partially hydrogenated vegetable fats, commonly known as trans fats (see page 129). It's also likely that they played a role in displacing the natural saturated and unsaturated fat these peoples had been used to eating.

Before the industrialisation of our food supply, humans obtained fat in their diet from:

1. **natural sources of saturated fats** from animal sources, such as butter, ghee, eggs, milk, cheese, cream, yoghurt,

meat and lard (pig fat) in addition to natural plant-based sources such as coconut oil, coconut butter and palm oil

2. **natural sources of monounsaturated fats**, including olive oil, suet or tallow (premium fat taken from around the kidneys of lamb or beef), and chicken or duck fat

3. **natural sources of polyunsaturated fats**, specifically those known as omega-3 from cold-water fatty fish such as salmon, mackerel, cod, herring, sardines and anchovies and from plant-based flaxseed oil and the common plant purslane; and omega-6, which is available in a large number of foods such as meats and plant foods, including nuts and seeds.

While these sources of fat (properly grown and prepared) appear to have played an important role in sustaining the physical and mental health of our ancestors for generations, fat consumption has been the source of extraordinary debate for several decades now. The debate has centred around claims that some fats are 'good' and are associated with good health and longevity while others are 'bad' and very harmful to human health.

Standard government dietary advice typically advises us to avoid the natural saturated fats we have eaten throughout human history in favour of polyunsaturated fats such as commercial 'heart healthy' margarines, and sunflower and safflower oils, in addition to fat from fatty fish such as salmon. The polyunsaturated fat component of this advice is now, however, rightly coming under scrutiny from diet sceptics. Polyunsaturated fatty acids come in two classes: omega-3 (e.g. alpha-linolenic acid) and omega-6 (e.g. linoleic acid). Linoleic acid occurs in high quantities in seed oils such as soybean oil (53 per cent), cottonseed oil (53 per cent), corn oil (57 per cent), sunflower oil (68 per cent) and safflower seed oil (78 per cent).

The most salient point to bear in mind is that when diet experts speak of 'bad' fat they are referring to saturated fat but when diet sceptics speak of 'bad' fat, they are referring to omega-6 fats. Although omega-6 fats are required for human health, they have flooded our food supply and consequently our bodies, throwing everything out of balance. Both omega-3 and omega-6 fatty acids also influence the expression of genes, particularly in people with gene variants that put them at greater risk of developing certain diseases.

The impact of omega-6

While humans require essential fatty acids such as polyunsaturated fatty acids for health, the major issue now being raised with regard to specific health problems is the ratio of omega-6 to omega-3 fats in our diet. Anthropological and epidemiological studies indicate that for millions of years humans and wild animals evolved on a diet with an omega-6 to omega-3 ratio of approximately 1:1. Over the last 150 years, however, the replacement in our diet of saturated fat and monounsaturated fat with seed oils such as the omega-6 heavy soybean oil commonly found in processed foods, has drastically altered this ratio to 15:1 or 20:1, although some estimates are substantially higher. The typical daily intake of omega-6 polyunsaturated fatty acids in the Western diet is thought to be in the vicinity of 12–17 grams, mostly derived from seed oils such as soybean oil.

In terms of public consumption, soybean oil has been the standout for decades and is today the second most consumed oil in the world after palm oil. (In Australia, canola oil and cottonseed make up 90 per cent of the seed oils produced.) Between 1909 and 1999, the estimated annual per capita consumption of soybean oil in the United States rose from 0.009 kilograms to 11.64 kilograms. While the amount of cottonseed oil in the American diet fell from a peak of 2 kilograms per capita annually in 1961 (level with soybean oil), from 1967 soybean oil commenced its breathtaking ascent to reach 11.64 kilograms per capita – far outstripping all other forms of fat.

Increase in Omega-6 Soybean Oil in the American Diet 1909–1999

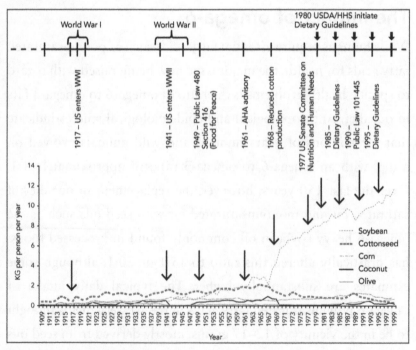

Source: Tanya L. Blasbalg et al.

Omega-6 and omega-3 content of common seed oils

Seed oil	Total omega-6 (milligrams per US tablespoon)	Total omega-3 (milligrams per US tablespoon)
Safflower	10,073	0
Grapeseed	9395	13.5
Wheatgerm	7398	932
Corn	7224	157
Walnut	7141	1404
Cottonseed	6953	27
Soybean	6807	917
Soybean/cottonseed (trans fat)	6116	378
Sunflower (normal)	5374	27
Margarine	4676	336
Canola	2610	1279
Sunflower (high-oleic)	505	26.9

Source: SELFNutritionData, nutritiondata.self.com

Omega-6 and omega-3 content of common saturated and monounsaturated fats

Saturated fat	Total omega-6 (milligrams per US tablespoon)	Total omega-3 (milligrams per US tablespoon)
Butter	382	44.1
Coconut oil	243	0
Olive oil	1318	103

Source: SELFNutritionData, nutritiondata.self.com

Omega-3 and omega-6 essential fatty acids are understood to metabolise to what are referred to as highly unsaturated fatty acids (HUFAs) which accumulate in tissues. Omega-3 HUFAs, eicosapentaenoic acid (EPA) and docosahexaenoic acid (DHA), are considered anti-inflammatory, as they are the precursors of anti-inflammatory eicosanoids that exhibit potent protective properties. These include containing cell damage, clearing infections and reducing pain associated with inflammation.

The major tissue HUFA from omega-6 is called arachidonic acid (AA), which in turn stimulates production of pro-inflammatory eicosanoids, potent agents that act on receptors found on or in nearly every cell and tissue in the body. One example is prostaglandins, which are involved in pain, swelling, fever, asthma attacks, blood clotting, menstrual cramps and labour, blood-pressure regulation and inflammation. The pro-inflammatory eicosanoids that result from AA are actively required in very small amounts, but when consistently produced in large amounts (stimulated by a diet heavy in omega-6) contribute to the chronic HUFA imbalance known as the arachidonic acid cascade.

This extraordinary imbalance of omega-6 in the diet is now coming under scrutiny as a 'promoter' of many prominent diseases related to a Western diet, such as cancer, infertility, mental health problems, skin conditions such as psoriasis, cardiovascular disease, osteoporosis, allergies and autoimmune diseases. Indeed, pharmaceutical companies, long aware of the negative impact of AA cascade overreactions, and of their propensity to impact nearly every tissue in the body, have spent billions of dollars developing and marketing products to suppress or control both the formation and action of the hormones that result from cascade reactions, without blocking the beneficial aspects of the cascade.

Aspirin, warfarin, Plavix and non-steroidal anti-inflammatory drugs (NSAIDs) act by slowing the formation of prostaglandins from arachidonic acid. NSAIDs are among the most commonly used drugs in the world, and more than 30 million people use them daily, but their side effects include gastrointestinal injury, kidney toxicity and cardiovascular events, particularly if they are taken with other drugs. Selective inhibitors were also developed to 'manage' the AA cascade, but the infamous heart drugs rofecoxib, also known as Vioxx, and celecoxib, known as Celebrex, unfortunately killed and maimed many trusting consumers in the process.

Current research looks to bring back aspirin as a cheap, readily obtainable drug for use in disease prevention. A large scale Australian study (which is part of a larger international study titled 'ASPREE') is now looking at the possibility that aspirin might be useful to treat or prevent a large array of conditions such as depression and inflammatory disorders including heart disease, type 2 diabetes, osteoporosis and other NCDs – symptoms of the Western diet and its chronic activation of the AA cascade. While this may prove to be an option, perhaps a transition to safer dietary fats, might be a better long-term goal.

In addition to the formation of eicosanoids, the AA cascade can also lead to an overreaction of the fragile endocannabinoid system, which is involved in appetite, mood, behaviour, fertility, and the regulation of the hormones insulin, leptin and ghrelin, which in turn are associated with obesity. The cannabinoid receptor CB1 is understood to be sensitive to omega-6 HUFA. But before exploring the full implications of this situation, we need to ask the obvious question of how we came to arrive here.

Trans fats

The story of fat has more twists and turns than an Agatha Christie novel, but to fully understand the issue we need to go back in history – again by 100 years. In 1911, a couple of very successful candle and soap makers called William Procter and James Gamble teamed up with a chemist with the idea of turning liquid cottonseed oil into a fat for human consumption, giving it the appetising name Crisco. Procter and Gamble used a process known as hydrogenation (forcing hydrogen through the cottonseed oil at high temperature) to keep the fat solid at room temperature. The end product was successfully marketed as a cheap and healthy shortening substitute through the 1920s onwards, via the sponsorship of radio programs known as 'soap operas' in addition to print advertising and Crisco-based cookbooks. By targeting advertising and promotion to mothers, Procter and Gamble were able to convince the primary cooks, caregivers and homemakers of the era that Crisco was superior in every way to traditional animal fats.

By the early 1940s, Procter and Gamble had perfected the art of partial hydrogenation of vegetable oil by blending their hydrogenated product with soybean oil to achieve a softer, less lard-like version. This new partially hydrogenated product had a high smoke point, making it attractive to the food and restaurant industry; took longer to go rancid, meaning it could be stored for long periods or transported to far-off places; and was cheaper, because the crushed soybeans required to make the oil were a by-product of the heavily subsidised animal-feed industry.

During the process, however, the basic structure of the fatty acids changed. This trans-fats-laden product was eventually consumed by millions in the form of margarine, packaged baked goods, fried fast foods and snack foods. By the mid-1960s the vast majority of America's fat consumption came from the blended cottonseed oil and soybean oil laced with trans fats.

WHAT ARE TRANS FATS?

As we saw on page 123, all unsaturated fatty acids contain what is known as a double carbon bond, but in natural fatty acids the attached hydrogen atoms are usually on the same side of the double bond, in what is called a cis (Latin for 'on this side of') arrangement. This creates a straight fatty acid molecule. In the hydrogenated fats, however, a significant proportion of the fatty acids ended up with their hydrogen atoms on opposite sides of the double bond, in what is known as a trans (Latin for 'on the other side') arrangement. This causes the fatty acid molecule to be bent.

While the American people blithely munched away on their trans-fat-filled treats, another American by the name of Ancel Keys was busy developing a theory; this would later inform the dietary guidelines that have led to the grim situation in which we now find ourselves. Keys, a professor of physiology, published a paper in 1953 known as 'The Six Countries Study'. In it, he hypothesised that the new scourge of the day, myocardial infarction, commonly known as a heart attack, was caused by too much fat in the diet. Keys's idea was supported by a diagram he had created showing a correlation between mortality from heart disease and 'fat calories' which was based upon fat consumption data from the Food and Agriculture Organization of the United Nations and death certificates from the World Health Organization.

Danish kidney specialist and medical sceptic Dr Uffe Ravnskov has since pointed out major flaws in Keys's 1953 paper, the most worrying being that although data was available for 22 countries, Keys only incorporated into his chart the six countries that supported his theory. For example, deaths from coronary heart disease in Finland were seven times those of Mexico, yet they both had the same amount of fat available to consume.

Despite the flaws, Keys concluded that cholesterol caused heart disease and the consumption of saturated fat raised cholesterol, therefore saturated-fat consumption caused heart disease and heart attacks. This conclusion became known as the diet–heart hypothesis. Once Keys appeared on the cover of *Time* magazine in 1961, foods containing natural saturated fats, such as eggs, butter, cheese, milk and cream, officially became 'dangerous' – a heart attack on a plate. In 1961, the American Heart Association (AHA) advised Americans to replace traditional saturated fats in their diet with polyunsaturated fats. Other Western countries, including Australia, soon followed suit.

Worried consumers now chose 'healthier' polyunsaturated margarine over butter and low-fat dairy instead of full-fat dairy, while eggs and cheese were no longer welcome at the breakfast table. In addition, public-health activists demanded that natural unsaturated fats, such as lard and beef tallow, be removed from restaurants and processed food. In the midst of the perfect storm of fat-bashing, edible-oil and processed-food manufacturers stepped up production of food offerings using oils high in trans fats, which could now be marketed as free from saturated fat and therefore a 'heart-healthy' option.

Trans fats were given another free kick during the 1980s, when the US Center for Science in the Public Interest (CSPI) applauded the use of these oils by food manufacturers and launched an all-out assault on food businesses that used beef fat and palm oil. The 1980s also saw the rise to national prominence of Phil Sokolof, the American cholesterol crusader who used his considerable private wealth to wage a public war on fat, fast-food restaurants and food manufacturers. Sokolof was a wealthy construction-supply magnate who, despite being a slim, exercising, non-smoker had his first heart attack at the age of 43. Sokolof used his own money to start the non-profit National Heart Savers Association and set about running expensive media campaigns warning citizens about the danger of cholesterol. To say that the well-meaning Sokolof wanted fat eradicated from the face of the earth would be an understatement – one of his campaigns urged Americans to switch from milk with 2 per cent fat to milk with no fat. In addition, he wanted food processors to remove natural fats such as coconut oil and palm oil from their products, and is credited with pushing McDonald's to stop cooking fries in traditional beef tallow. Between Keys's not so scientific 'evidence', the CSPI's endorsement and Sokolof's media campaign, the embedding of omega-6 fats heavy in trans fats in the Western diet became a shoo-in.

In 1990, an important study was published in the *New England Journal of Medicine*. The authors, Ronald Mensink and Martijn Katan, noting that trans fats were being consumed in large amounts by the public, decided to place 59 healthy men and women between the ages of nineteen and 57 on three diets that were exactly the same apart from a slight difference in fatty acid profile – one group ate largely cis polyunsaturated oleic acid (sunflower oil), the second oleic acid high in trans fats, and the third saturated fatty acids. The results of the study confirmed other reports that trans fatty acids drove up cholesterol levels more than oleic acid and saturated fatty acids. The more alarming finding, however, was that trans fatty acids were able to raise 'bad' cholesterol, low-density lipoprotein (LDL), and lower 'good' cholesterol, high-density lipoprotein (HDL), in the blood of the participants.

Needless to say, a series of bunfights between stakeholders ensued, and consumers wondered whether they had been shunted from the frying pan into the fire. The CSPI performed a back-flip, pursuing an aggressive campaign to have trans fats labelled, a process that took twelve years but enabled manufacturers to develop replacement fats. Studies linking trans fats to human disease continued to appear, and after more than two decades of bad news, the US Food and Drug Administration (FDA) in 2013 issued a preliminary notice that trans fats are not 'generally recognised as safe', and in June 2015 gave industry a three-year deadline to remove them from all processed foods. In Australia, there are no labelling laws regarding trans fats, but the amounts in our food are very low (averaging 0.5 per cent of our daily energy intake) and the majority are naturally occurring rather than manufactured.

While the trans fats debacle appears to be coming to an end, the notion that there is today a clear public understanding or consensus on dietary fat consumption would be premature – as would any delusions that the processed-food industry has made a transition to anything safer. The diet–heart hypothesis still appears to be the dominant paradigm among the diet experts, even when new information emerges, while heart disease continues to be the leading cause of death not just in Australia, but the world.

Highly unsaturated fatty acids

The official advice to replace saturated fat with unsaturated fat piqued the interest of one William Lands, a lipid biochemist at the University of Michigan Medical School, who wondered by what exact mechanism saturated fat could be universally (and officially) declared 'bad' while monounsaturated and polyunsaturated fats were declared 'good'. After all, as an expert in fats, Lands knew that healthy human tissues constantly make both saturated and unsaturated fats from foods. Saturated fats make up half the fatty acids in cell membranes, and saturated fatty acids range in length from twelve to 24 carbons, making it difficult to identify which of them were the silent killers. Lands noted that several population groups consumed diets high in coconut and palm oil, yet were not dying of heart disease, while human breastmilk appears designed to ensure the baby absorbs saturated fat above all other available fatty acids. Moreover, epidemiologists had long been aware that fish-loving Mediterranean and Japanese populations were less susceptible to ischaemic heart disease than Americans. Non-Westernised people from Greenland were even less susceptible to heart disease than the Japanese.

Born in 1930, Professor Lands has been ringside at the fat fight for decades. To date, Lands, one of the world's 1000 most cited scientists, has been unable to identify a definite causal mechanism or mediator of harm attributable to 'toxic' saturated fat and continues to be bewildered at the insistence by official diet committees that people actively consume higher levels of omega-6 fats than are required for health. What Lands also understands, however, is that polyunsaturated fatty acids and in particular the longer-chain twenty- and 22-carbon HUFAs, selectively accumulate in tissues, and that potent pro-inflammatory eicosanoids are consequently formed. The HUFAs become incorporated into hormones such as prostaglandins, which play a role in inflammation, thrombosis, atherosclerosis, asthma, arthritis, cancer, dementia and cardiovascular disease. These HUFAs can be either omega-3 or omega-6, but food choices favouring greater omega-3 consumption and a dramatic reduction in omega-6 consumption can go a long way to ameliorating the negative effects of high HUFA levels in body tissues.

With his knowledge of the importance of tissue HUFA in human health, Lands analysed the food habits of several ethnic groups and observed that coronary heart disease rates in certain populations were associated with the ratio of omega-6 to omega-3 HUFAs in tissues. For example, fish-eating people from Greenland and Japan (both populations with historically low mortality from heart disease) have omega-6 tissue HUFA levels at between 20–40 per cent of total HUFA while in American and Quebec urban populations these are closer to 80 per cent. Deaths from heart disease are many times higher in America and urban Quebec, a situation that becomes very predictable in populations that make the transition to the Western, omega-6-heavy diet.

In an effort to help people correct their own tissue HUFA levels, Lands created an online tool called www.efaeducation.org. This offers information to help people create a personal diet plan to 'Nix6 and Eat3'; links to accessing a finger-prick blood test that measures your current HUFA balance from your current diet; and apps that help you work out which foods will help you achieve a better HUFA balance and which foods to eliminate from your diet.

Re-evaluation of old data

While Lands' online tool is helpful for people who would like to improve their health, research groups continue to unravel the mystery of why we had to have the misguided war on saturated fat in the first place. In 2013, a group of researchers from the NIH and University of Carolina decided to take a second look at previously unpublished data collected during the famous Sydney Diet Heart Study. This single-blinded, parallel-group, randomised controlled trial conducted from 1966 to 1973 involved 458 men aged 30–59 who had had a recent coronary event. The aim of the study was to lower serum cholesterol in the diet by replacing traditional saturated fats with safflower oil rich in linoleic acid (omega-6). Controls made no any changes to their diet. The researchers found that while the increased consumption of linoleic acid significantly reduced blood cholesterol, the intervention group demonstrated increased rates of death not just from all causes, but also from cardiovascular disease and coronary heart disease.

Still curious, the same group of researchers subsequently decided to reanalyse unpublished data from the Minnesota Coronary Experiment (MCE), a double-blind randomised controlled trial involving 9423 men and women aged twenty to 97 conducted from 1968 to 1973. This re-analysis was published in the *British Medical Journal* in April 2016. The MCE, conducted by Ancel Keys and Ivan Frantz, is considered to be the largest and most tightly controlled dietary study ever undertaken involving lowering cholesterol by replacing saturated fat with linoleic acid. The aim of the study was to test whether replacement of saturated fat from traditional dietary sources with seed oil rich in omega-6 linoleic acid (in this case corn oil) lowers blood cholesterol levels and consequently the rate of coronary heart disease and death.

Unlike the Sydney Diet Heart Study, the MCE is the only study of its type to undertake post-mortem evaluation of hardening of the arteries and potential for heart attack of almost 300 participants. Although only 149 of the autopsy files were recovered by the researchers conducting the reanalysis, who stressed that the findings should be interpreted with due caution given the incomplete files, they revealed that within the autopsy cohort, 31 out of 76 participants from the linoleic acid group had at least one heart attack compared with just sixteen out of 73 participants from the control (saturated fat) group. In addition, the authors could find no association between blood cholesterol levels and heart attack or hardening of the arteries. The authors note that the seed oil diet did reduce blood cholesterol in the patients but this had no positive effect on heart disease. In fact, patients who lowered their cholesterol suffered more heart-related deaths than those who didn't, particularly in the over-64 age group.

Like Bill Lands, the authors queried the wisdom of the current dietary recommendations to replace saturated fat with omega-6-heavy vegetable oil. Why the full results of the Minnesota trial were never published remains a mystery we will probably never solve, particularly in light of the fact that both Keys and Frantz are now deceased.

Endocannabinoids

In my discussion of the omega-6-driven AA cascade (see page 128), I mentioned the endocannabinoid system. While most people would not have heard of this system, they would definitely have heard of the catalyst for its discovery – cannabis.

The cannabis plant has been used as medicine since ancient times. The Chinese emperor Shen-nung (c. 2000 BC) noted in an ancient work called *Pen-ts'ao Ching* that, among other effects, cannabis 'undoes rheumatism'. Rheumatoid arthritis, considered to be an autoimmune disease, appears to have affected Weston Price's study subjects after consumption of store foods. It's now understood to involve infiltration of immune cells into the synovial membrane between joints, as well as chronic inflammation. Eicosanoids from the AA cascade play a role in the ongoing destruction of cartilage and bone. Eicosapentaenoic acid from omega-3 sources, however, decreases production of AA-derived eicosanoids and decreases the inflammatory response.

Cannabis is mentioned in the Zoroastrian faith's Sacred Book of Knowledge (600–1000 BC), and cannabis seeds have been found inside a 3000-year-old Siberian burial mound. The Jewish religious scholar, philosopher and physician Maimonides, who lived in the twelfth century, noted that cannabis was a commonly used medical drug. Arabic records from the fifteenth century tell of the epileptic son of the chamberlain of the Caliphate Council in Baghdad being prescribed hashish by a doctor, which cured him of the epilepsy on the condition that he smoke it for the rest of his life. Both the ancient Chinese and Greeks used cannabis to treat multiple-sclerosis-like symptoms such as muscle spasms and tremors. For the vast expanse of history, cannabis was legal and used around the world by herbalists, shamans and healers in tinctures. By 1851, 'tincture of cannabis' was listed in the US pharmacopoeia and routinely used by American doctors for treating ailments.

Despite the non-controversial use of the cannabis plant industrially (to produce hemp) and medicinally, a 'war' on cannabis began in earnest with the introduction in the United States of the Marihuana Tax Act of 1937. The new tax on cannabis was strongly opposed by the American Medical Association, as it affected a doctor's ability to prescribe medicinal cannabis, and to manufacture or sell the tinctures. The tax was drafted by one Harry Anslinger – nephew-in-law of banker, industrialist, financial backer of the DuPont chemical family interests, United States Secretary of the Treasury Andrew W. Mellon. Anslinger had been appointed by Mellon to head the Federal Bureau of Narcotics in 1930.

Perhaps the most thoroughly researched book on the machinations behind the scheme to outlaw all cannabis use is *Hemp – American History Revisited: The Plant with a Divided History* by Robert Deitch, which details a sordid history featuring the usual cast of monopolists from the oil, petrochemical, newspaper publishing and banking industries, and their role in wiping medical and industrial cannabis from the landscape. So sustained and successful was the war on cannabis that in 1970, with no scientific evidence to support the claim, President Richard Nixon declared cannabis a Schedule 1 drug (the same category as heroin) with no accepted medicinal use (a decision reaffirmed by the US Drug Enforcement Agency in 2016).

In 1963 in Israel, a renegade organic chemist by the name of Raphael Mechoulam – a fascinating man whose story was told in the 2015 documentary *The Scientist* – decided to study the plant's chemical composition and eventually identified an array of substances, including the psychoactive compounds delta-9-tetrahydrocannabinol (THC) and cannabidiol (CBD). Further research in the late 1980s and early 1990s (much of it funded by the US NIH using taxpayer money) revealed the existence of two cannabinoid receptors in humans. The first was CB1, which is related to the THC effects of cannabis and expressed in the brain, central nervous system, gut and peripheral tissues; and CB2, which likely forms part of a protective system in the human body (particularly in the brain) and is expressed in the immune, blood and brain cells. Both receptors are broadly distributed in the human body and found in the brain, foetal membranes, pituitary gland, breasts, reproductive tissues, endothelial cells, placenta, white blood cells and eye.

Assuming that God in his wisdom did not give us cannabinoid receptors so we could all become stoners, Mechoulam and his team went in search of the other part of the puzzle – the natural molecules found in the human body that would bind to the receptors. In 1992 the group isolated a molecule that binds to the same brain receptor as THC and named it anandamide (also known as N-arachidonoylethanolamine or AEA), based on the Sanskrit word *ananda* for 'supreme joy' or 'bliss'. Research published in 2016 revealed that the well-known 'runner's high' experienced by long-distance athletes may not be due to endorphins as first thought, as they are too large to cross the blood–brain barrier, but rather to anandamide, levels of which increase in the bloodstream after 30 minutes of exercise.

The group later discovered the second molecule, 2-Arachidonoyl glycerol (2-AG) in the gut of a dog around the same time a Japanese group found it in the human brain. Together, the two cannabinoid receptors (CB1 and CB2) and the two endocannabinoids (anandamide and 2-AG) and their enzymes form the endocannabinoid system. Research in this field has exploded in recent times.

Infertility

Studies have now emerged linking dysregulation of the endocannabinoid system to virtually all classes of human disease. Receptors have been detected in almost all components of the reproductive system and at all stages of fertilisation and foetal development. Scientists know that in order for an egg to travel into the uterus and an embryo to successfully implant itself on the uterine wall, CB1 receptor expression must be balanced.

Excessive CB1 expression is involved in miscarriage and infertility, while low CB1 is found in ectopic pregnancy. In the developing foetus, the ECS is involved in the structural and functional development of the nervous system. Once the baby is born, CB1 is involved in initiating breastfeeding which is essential to the baby's ability to thrive. Anandamide, the lipid signalling molecule that activates CB1, has even been referred to as possibly the 'guardian angel of reproduction'. Balanced endocannabinoid signalling appears to be critical to successful reproduction, which is why marijuana exposure in both men and women is understood to be involved with infertility and with adverse events during pregnancy.

Endocannabinoids are intimately connected to dietary fatty acid consumption, because both anandamide and 2-AG are derivatives of the AA cascade, production of which is stimulated by omega-6 fats from such sources as soybean, corn, cottonseed, safflower and sunflower seed oil. According to researchers, dietary fats are the *only* source of fatty acids required for synthesis of endocannabinoids, so it naturally begs the question whether chronic consumption of omega-6 fats via the processed food supply might modulate circulating endocannabinoid levels and lead to negative health effects, including the observed dramatic increase in fertility problems.

Depression, anxiety and behavioural problems

Fertility problems are merely the beginning of a number of health issues exploding in the West that are linked to a 'swamped' endocannabinoid signalling system. According to the World Health Organization, anxiety and depression are leading contributors to the global burden of disease, depression alone affecting 350 million people worldwide. Depression and anxiety among young people, particularly women, are deemed to be a growing problem, and suicide is today the second leading cause of death globally in the fifteen to 29 age bracket. While evidence suggests that many people are being misdiagnosed and wrongly medicated for depression, the problem is considered to be a growing global issue. So where does fat fit in?

Problems with CB1 receptors have been linked to various psychiatric, neurological and neurodevelopmental disorders. The endocannabinoid system is abundantly expressed in the brain and central nervous system, and broadly distributed throughout the body. The CB1 receptor is considered to be the most plentiful neurotransmitter receptor in the brain and the central nervous system, where its activity controls brain development, learning, memory, motor behaviour, appetite regulation, body temperature, inflammation and pain perception. In addition, the distribution of CB1 receptors appears to be highly relevant; receptors located on neurons (nerve cells) where gamma-aminobutyric acid (GABA) is the neurotransmitter, for example, have been shown to control appetite, 'runner's high', drug addiction, learning and memory. CB1 receptors located on neurons where glutamate is the neurotransmitter can control anxiety, phobia, fear memories, habituation, taste, neuroprotection and social behaviours. CB1 receptors on neurons where serotonin is the neurotransmitter can regulate emotional responses to social stress.

The endocannabinoid system is understood to be vital in

mediating normal adolescent behaviour due to its influence on neurological processes that intensify during the transition from child to adult. The adolescent brain is uniquely susceptible to depressive disorders; moodiness; impulsivity; and high-risk, reward and novelty-seeking behaviours. It's also especially susceptible to drug abuse. While detailed mechanisms under-pinning adolescent brain development are not fully understood, scientists are now examining the role of expression of the CB1 receptor, which increases during adolescence. Scientists have also found that omega-3 deficiency (likely generated through an excess of omega-6 and the AA cascade) leads to learning, cognitive, attention and behavioural problems in children and young people.

Researchers from the Avon Longitudinal Study of Parents and Children (ALSPAC) in Bristol, United Kingdom, found that babies born to mothers who consumed more than 340 grams of fish (which is high in omega-3) per week produced children who scored higher on communication and verbal IQ scores than mothers who either did not consume fish or consumed less than 340 grams per week. In a separate randomised, double-blind, placebo-controlled, stratified, parallel-group trial, children aged eight to sixteen were given 1 gram per day of omega-3 or a placebo for six months. The researchers found that the omega-3 group exhibited a 42–68 per cent reduction in reported antisocial and aggressive behaviour, which extended a full six months beyond the trial. Moreover, parents of children in the treatment group found their own behaviour improved as they were suddenly parenting calmer children, which improved their own stress levels.

Multiple sclerosis and gastrointestinal diseases

Many human cells contain small membrane-bound bodies called mitochondria, which have their own DNA and provide the cell with energy. CB1 receptors are located on both cell membranes and mitochondrial membranes, and cannabinoids (anandamide and 2-AG) can alter mitochondrial function. Mitochondrial dysfunction is a feature of many chronic diseases, including muscle wastage and movement disorders. Dr Terry Wahls, who reversed her secondary progressive multiple sclerosis symptoms, has referred to her illness as a mitochondrial disease. She credited supplementation with omega-3 fatty acids and micronutrients as instrumental to her recovery.

Researchers from the Endocannabinoid Research Group in Naples and the Eicosanoid and Lipid Research Division at the Free University Berlin found that anandamide levels are significantly higher in intestinal biopsies of people with active coeliac disease than non-coeliac sufferers, an observation that also applied to experimental models of ulcerative colitis and diverticular disease. Moreover, anandamide levels returned to normal on a gluten-free diet. The up-regulation of anandamide was accompanied by an up-regulation of CB1 receptors, indicating that anandamide is heavily involved in gastrointestinal inflammatory diseases.

The immune system

The endocannabinoid system is also involved in modula-tion of the immune response and inflammatory reactions, and may play a role in homeostasis (balancing) of the immune system. Endocannabinoids modulate the proliferation of T- and B-lymphocytes (immune cells) and programmed cell death, as well as activation of immune cells in response to inflammation caused by cytokines (see page 37). Antibody-producing B-lymphocytes have also been shown to have many CB2 receptors. Studies have shown that endocannabinoids modulate the formation of antibodies to keep them in balance. It's understood that eicosanoid signalling facilitates cross-talk between endocannabinoid signalling and regulation of the immune system. Tissue levels of endocannabinoids have been shown to be dependent on gender and hormonal cycles, which may explain why women are so prone to immune system dysfunction and autoimmune diseases, particularly at times of peak hormonal changes, such as adolescence and menopause.

Bone health

Weston Price's research subjects experienced bone problems once they started consuming (or were born to parents consuming) store foods including seed oil. It turns out that endocannabinoid signalling is also involved in the bone-remodelling process. Both anandamide and 2-AG are produced in bone cells in similar levels to those in brain cells. Mice that lack CB2 receptors show age-related loss of bone density similar to postmenopausal osteoporosis in women, while in humans differences in the genes involved with CB2 formation can lead to low bone mass and osteoporosis. The effect of the endocannabinoid system on bones can be seen in the babies of women who used marijuana while pregnant; these babies have a reduced foetal growth rate, reduced birth weight, reduced head circumference and shorter stature. Researchers note that endocannabinoid signalling regulates bone elongation and remodelling by modulating the formation of bone cells and communication between them.

Obesity

Diets high in linoleic acid from such sources as soybean oil have been found to promote obesity and are linked to increased fasting blood glucose, fasting blood insulin and insulin resistance. Obese and overweight people have been found to have poorly regulated endocannabinoids in peripheral tissues, which interferes with glucose and fat metabolism. Elevated endocannabinoid levels have been found in the saliva of fasting insulin-resistant people, and these levels were positively correlated with blood-insulin concentrations. Circulating 2-AG levels are higher in obese people, and increased 2-AG is also associated with higher body mass index, waist circumference and abdominal fat. Rimonabant, an anti-obesity drug, worked by blocking CB1 receptors, but was withdrawn due to side effects including depression, eating disorders and suicide risk. Because anandamide signalling is involved with so many systems and processes in the body, drugs affecting it can produce a wide range of unwanted and potentially dangerous side effects.

Researchers have hypothesised that elevated levels of endocannabinoid may lead people to overconsume carbohydrate-rich food and unsaturated fats such as seed oils. Is the famous 'bliss point' merely describing the ability of junk food to activate our own built-in anandamide 'high'? Interestingly, endocannabinoids have been detected in 'addictive' foods such as chocolate, in addition to milk, hazelnuts, soybeans and millet.

Attempts at change

It would appear that health problems associated with excessive omega-6 intake (sometimes referred to as dietary omega-3 deficiency syndrome) is not new knowledge to some. In 2012, a group of science and policy gurus met at the Rockefeller Foundation's Bellagio Center at Lake Como to discuss, among other things, substances in the diet that were negatively affecting the health of the population, particularly children. Tying for first place were sugary soft drinks (referred to as an insidious health threat akin to cigarette smoking), and the overabundance of omega-6 fatty acids and deficiency of omega-3 fatty acids in the food supply. Apart from health warnings on soft drinks, the authors recommended that the ratio of omega-6 to omega-3 fatty acids should be decreased and that governments should educate or intervene to ensure populations switch from oils high in omega-6 to those high in omega-3 and to monounsaturated oils such as olive oil. In addition, the American Psychiatric Society has recommended a daily minimum of 1 gram of omega-3 for adults with certain psychiatric conditions, but strangely nothing for youth, while the 2010 *Dietary Guidelines for Americans* advised seafood two to three times per week for children.

In 2014, the American Society for Nutrition, a group (supported by companies including Monsanto, McDonald's, Cargill, Coca-Cola, PepsiCo, Pfizer, Kellogg Company, the Sugar Association, Unilever and Tate & Lyle – you get the picture) that wishes to be seen as the 'trusted global authority' on nutrition, issued a scientific statement titled 'Processed foods: contributions to nutrition'. While the paper was mostly a pro-processed-food manifesto, it did clearly state that the ratio of omega-6 to omega-3 ratio is too high. It also noted that solving the problem was difficult given that fish, a good source of omega-3, is unsustainable (a position disputed by some experts in the field) so other solutions such as nanotechnology might be preferred. The 100-year feeding experiment continues.

While more research into the impact of processed food on both the AA cascade and endocannabinoid system, and its impact on human health is clearly necessary, as individual consumers we can solve the problem of too much omega-6 fats in our diet simply by eating real food as nature intended. As processed foods are the major vector by which an oversupply of omega-6 enters our system, a simple diet of low-omega-6 unprocessed foods with fats drawn from traditional sources, alongside greater intake of fish or fish oil, is a step in the right direction. Perhaps Jesus, whose symbol was the fish, was trying to tell us something after all.

6

Can sugar make us sick?

With its inescapable early ties to the Trans-Atlantic slave trade and the abolitionist movement, the bittersweet history of sugar is shameful and violent. Its role in the destruction of Weston Price's indigenous research subjects was but another shocking milestone in sugar's less than wholesome march through time.

Sugar and slavery

Once upon a time sugar was so rare it was considered, alongside cardamom and nutmeg, to be a luxury spice available for consumption only by the European and British elite. Legend has it that in 1598 a German traveller noted the black teeth of Queen Elizabeth I, referring to the problem as a 'defect the English seem subject to have from their too great use of sugar'. So hooked did the aristocracy become on the substance that expedition parties were sent forth into the world to discover tropical locations that could support sugar plantations and assure a steady supply of sugar to the teacups of the upper classes.

As more islands and territories were discovered, colonised and razed to make way for increased sugar production, the search for cheap labour began in earnest. When indigenous populations initially forced to work the fields died from disease, exhaustion or accident in the hot and dangerous conditions, plantation owners felt they had little choice but to import labour to keep up with sugar demand. The labour shipments came to be known as the Trans-Atlantic slave trade.

While the highly sanitised Hollywood depiction of African slavery typically portrays robust people toiling on quaint cotton plantations in South Carolina or Georgia, for the men, women and children dragged from their African villages and force-marched for days or weeks to the port towns of the Slave Coast along the Bight of Benin in West Africa, the experience of slavery was markedly different.

Loaded onto seagoing vessels roughly 30 metres long, slaves were chained in cramped coffin-sized rows in dark, filthy, airless ship holds and transported across lurching Atlantic seas to the New World to cultivate sugar cane by hand. Records from the time indicate that more than 11 million slaves embarked upon the infamous Middle Passage journey between the West Coast of Africa and the Americas, and around 9.6 million survived. More than two-thirds of this tragic human cargo was destined for life on the sugar plantations.

For those who survived the Middle Passage, life in the British West Indies was extremely brutal, and slaves were effectively worked to death. By the time slavery was abolished in the United States in 1865, the initial 500,000 slave population had grown to around 4 million. The slave numbers in the British West Indies provide a stark contrast, dwindling from 2 million slaves originally sent there to a population of around 670,000 by the time slavery was abolished. One of the main reasons the population could not naturally sustain itself or even increase was rampant infertility among the African women due to poor health.

Meanwhile in Britain, the most basic laws of supply and demand enabled sugar prices to fall and the addiction to spread to the homes of the middle classes. Prices and barriers to trade continued to drop, enabling sugar not just to become available to the poor, but a staple of their diet. Indeed, the consumption of sugar in Britain rose from around 2 kilograms per year in 1700 to around 45 kilograms per year by the late twentieth century.

As report after report of the unmerciful and murderous conditions endured by slaves working the plantations in the British West Indies made its way back to British society, a growing unease began to manifest itself among the consuming population. People suddenly refused to purchase 'slave-grown sugar' in protest at the outrageous treatment of slaves. In what might be considered the first recorded consumer backlash against unethical business practices, the whispers surrounding the human cost of sugar eventually rose to the scream that would catapult fledgling notions of human rights and consumer activism to centre stage.

On 27 May 1787, a group of twelve average and unassuming men met at a printing shop at 2 George Yard, London. There, they set about organising a grassroots citizen's movement that would challenge and ultimately defeat the might of the extremely wealthy and powerful British elites for whom slave trading was a cornerstone of mercantile interests. Horrified by what they had learned about slavery and the slave trade, they set about educating the citizenry on the subject. In a move that until then had been without precedent, the people began petitioning Parliament to end Britain's role in slave trading, and they kept the issue alive until the House of Commons passed the first law banning the slave trade in 1807.

The British abolitionists set themselves the extraordinary and seemingly impossible task of putting an end to the 'enormous evil' of slavery, a firmly entrenched practice that had for thousands of years been considered the norm by ruling classes the world over. It may have taken 50 years of advocacy to finally pass anti-slavery laws in Britain, but the pivotal role of sugar in ending forced servitude might seem paradoxical. Sadly, in little over 100 years, sugar would come to be associated with a new form of slavery, albeit of the biochemical kind, one that binds us not to the plantation, but to poor health and disability.

WHAT IS SUGAR?

Sugar, or more precisely sugars, are sweet soluble carbohydrates with short carbon chains (or rings). These can be monosaccharides (single or simple sugars), disaccharides (double sugars) or oligosaccharides (sugars with six to ten simple sugars). The most common simple sugars are glucose (also known as dextrose), fructose and galactose. The sugar we are most familiar with – table sugar or sucrose – is a disaccharide, made up of one glucose molecule bound to one fructose molecule. Other disaccharides include lactose (milk sugar), which is a combination of glucose and galactose, and maltose, which is a combination of two glucose molecules. Oligosaccharides occur naturally in fruits and vegetables.

John Yudkin and the sugar problem

If you really want to understand what foods and chemicals do to your body, forget the marketing brochure and ask a very experienced (and preferably independent) biochemist instead. It's their job to study and understand the chemical processes involved in all basic life functions. Through their work they bring new insight into the effects of foods and chemicals (synthetic and naturally occurring) on living cells and organisms. They understand the concept of feedback the same way a computer programmer understands the concept of 'garbage in, garbage out'.

It was a British biochemist called John Yudkin who first raised the idea of negative health implications surrounding sugar in the diet back in 1972 with his book *Pure, White and Deadly: How Sugar Is Killing Us and What We Can Do to Stop it.*

Yudkin, the founder of the Nutrition Department at the University of London's Queen Elizabeth College, had completed a number of studies regarding the effects of sugar and carbohydrate consumption on both animals and humans. His sugar research identified correlations between sugar consumption and obesity, tooth decay, heart disease and diabetes, but as scientists and industry shills alike are always quick to point out, correlation does not imply causation.

It was his stance regarding heart disease that famously drew him into battle with Ancel Keys, the American physiologist whose ultimately flawed 'Six Countries Study' connected diets high in animal fats with high cholesterol and heart disease. In 1961 Keys had appeared on the cover of *Time* magazine, and the accompanying article, which asserted that dietary saturated fats such as butter and lard caused clogged arteries and heart disease, set off the 'war on saturated fat'. While the particulars of this battle between Keys and Yudkin have been recorded in books and documentaries over many years, the fact that obesity, diabetes and cancer have continued to rise to alarming levels means that sugar, refined grains and seed oils in particular have again come under the microscope.

When Yudkin's book was published in 1972, he was possessed of what amounted to signposts. He had found, for example, that when rats ate sugar, their blood-triglyceride (fat) levels increased to a great extent, whereas their blood-cholesterol levels did not. He found that sugar-fed rats developed an enlarged liver and adrenal glands, and exhibited abnormalities in how their pancreas made insulin. In addition, the aortas of sugar-fed rats contained substantially increased amounts of cholesterol and triglycerides. In human studies, Yudkin found that high-sugar diets could result in a rise in triglycerides, blood cholesterol, insulin and platelet stickiness (indicating a propensity to form dangerous blood clots), but he conceded that genetics and complex metabolic processes were possibly involved in his varying results.

Yudkin never asserted that particular diseases were 'caused' by sugar, and he made the point that genetics and environment were the major determinants of disease development. But his research put forward the idea that sugar was likely one of the chief environmental factors at play.

More than 40 years after the Keys–Yudkin stoush took place, the US government published the *Report of the 2015 Dietary Guidelines Advisory Committee*. The introduction to this report immediately highlighted the fact that half of all American adults (117 million people) have one or more preventable chronic diseases – such as cardiovascular disease, hypertension, type 2 diabetes and diet-related cancers – that are a result of poor diet and lack of movement. The introduction noted that more than two-thirds of US adults and nearly one-third of children and young people are overweight or obese. When the official US dietary guidelines were first published in 1980, 5.6 million Americans had been diagnosed with diabetes. At the time of publishing the 2015 guidelines, more than 29.1 million Americans or 9.3 per cent of the population had been diagnosed, and a further 86 million Americans aged twenty and above had been diagnosed as pre-diabetic, an increase of 7 million in just two years.

The introduction also noted that these shocking health problems have persisted for decades and placed enormous financial pressure on US health care, and recommended that Americans reconsider their diet and eat real foods such as vegetables, fruits, diary and wholegrains. The authors also made one startling admission: population intake 'is too high for refined grains and added sugars'.

Added sugars in the diet have become the latest battleground between nutritionists, doctors, dietitians, journalists, bloggers, documentary filmmakers, biochemists, lobbyists and industry spokespeople. Anti-sugar advocates argue that sugar is effectively a toxin that when consumed in even moderate amounts can send our chemistry off balance, resulting in insulin resistance, obesity, metabolic syndrome, type 2 diabetes, damaged organs and tissues, cancer and cardiovascular disease. Critics draw the crowd's attention to 'premature claims', 'insufficient evidence', 'poorly understood mechanisms' and 'general misconceptions' surrounding the issue. And all the while, growing numbers of concerned consumers – tired of 'waiting for the science to ripen' – are quietly removing sugars, excess carbohydrate and processed seed oils from their diets, and experiencing remission from the symptoms of some of these conditions.

The immune system

One of the most interesting aspects of Weston Price's study is his observation of increased susceptibility of indigenous groups to pathogens such as viruses, bacteria and yeasts after consumption of 'store foods', and their return to health (even from diseases such as tuberculosis, an infection caused by the bacterium *Mycobacterium tuberculosis*) upon resuming their traditional diet. Might sugar have played a role in lowering their immune response to pathogens? And if so, can we take a lesson from them and better protect our own health from pathogens by avoiding added sugar?

In Chapter 4 I discussed a protein called mannose-binding lectin (MBL) and its role in recognising and destroying viruses, bacteria and yeasts. People who suffer from chronic infections may have dysfunctional or low levels of MBL linked to genetic variations, but could another factor be at play? A group of immunology and gastroenterology researchers from Harvard Medical

School decided to look at how dietary sugars affect human disease and immune function. Already aware that dietary sugar (but not starch) effectively diminishes the ability of white blood cells called phagocytes to engulf and destroy bacteria (in a process called phagocytosis, literally 'devouring cells'), the researchers were interested in finding out whether sugar could play a role in inhibiting the biological functions of MBL.

The study found that dietary fructose down-regulated MBL mechanisms against the viral pathogen influenza A and the bacterial pathogen *Staphylococcus aureus* by reducing MBL-induced phagocytosis. The researchers concluded that dietary sugars, in particular fructose, negatively impact the innate immune response against both viruses and bacteria. This is an important finding given our high levels of sugar consumption and the tendency of type 2 diabetes patients to develop infections. The authors speculate that high levels of sugar consumption could mimic MBL deficiency, leaving both the healthy and the sick at risk of increased susceptibility to infection.

Tooth decay

Because Weston Price was a dentist, he was particularly interested in the oral health of the populations he visited. Price made many references to the role of sugar in the destruction of teeth, and the terrible toll it was taking on the populations he studied, particularly in light of the lack of proper dental care available to them. It's now known that dental caries (tooth decay) can be caused by the colonisation of teeth with cariogenic or caries-inducing bacteria, and that sucrose is the most cariogenic sugar.

Under conditions of high or constant sugar consumption, these bacteria form dental plaques and metabolise the sugar into organic acids. These acids lower the pH of the plaque and dissolve the dental enamel. Chronically low pH leads to development of caries through constant demineralisation. Removal of sugar from the diet and regularly cleaning the teeth can help the remineralisation process. Many epidemiological studies conducted in developing nations have demonstrated a rise in dental caries in parallel with a rise in sugar consumption, mirroring Weston Price's observations.

Dental caries is still a major health problem around the world. The Global Burden of Diseases Study 2013 noted 200 million cases of tooth pain attributed to dental caries. In Britain alone, almost 26,000 general anaesthetics are given to children between the ages of five to nine each year to have teeth removed due to sugar damage. In some centres, children must wait up to a year for the procedure, due to the extraordinary backlog of cases.

In an interesting aside regarding the role of the sugar industry in censoring the risks associated with consumption, a recently discovered cache of internal sugar-industry documents from the years 1959–71 revealed that America's publicly funded NIH had worked closely with industry to align federal US research projects with industry interests in the area of children's tooth decay. Independent analysis of the archive of 319 industry documents stored at the University of Illinois revealed that both the dental community and sugar industry worked on developing research approaches that promoted ways of reducing tooth decay in American children without sugar reduction in processed foods. To this end, a new vaccine was proposed against the bacteria causing tooth decay as well as adding enzymes to processed foods that would break up dental plaques. Perhaps most damning was the fact that 78 per cent of a report submitted to the US National Institute of Dental Research (NIDR) by the sugar industry was slotted directly into the NIDR's initial request for research proposals for the National Caries Program (NCP) and 'research that could have been harmful to sugar industry interests ... was omitted from [the research] priorities identified at the NCP'.

The independent researchers noted that even today the sugar industry's position is to focus attention on *anything* but the sugar, pushing fluoride toothpaste and dental sealants over restricted consumption. In addition, they lament the lost opportunity to protect children from more than just tooth decay.

Metabolic syndrome

Like many of us living in developed nations, many indigenous groups now suffer under the yoke of metabolic syndrome and type 2 diabetes. Sugar's connection to metabolic syndrome has placed it firmly in the spotlight again. Metabolic syndrome was once known as syndrome X, a term that has been around for almost 30 years. It was coined by endocrinologist Gerald M. Reaven at the 1988 Banting Lecture, an annual research presentation given by experts in diabetes (named for Frederick Banting, who won the 1923 Nobel Prize in medicine for his discovery of insulin).

Reaven, who has been called the 'father of insulin resistance', first established its role in human disease and in type 2 diabetes. He has also been credited with discovering the links between insulin resistance (and compensatory high blood insulin) and the development of a 'complex' of chronic-disease symptoms that are today referred to as metabolic syndrome.

Today the official metabolic syndrome 'complex' includes elevated blood pressure, elevated fasting glucose, abdominal obesity and dyslipidemia (elevated triglycerides and lowered HDL cholesterol), a combination that may lead to type 2 diabetes as well as cardiovascular disease. Reaven also noted that simply being obese was not a reliable indicator of metabolic syndrome; many people who are thin or of normal weight also develop insulin resistance, a situation commonly described as TOFI – thin on the outside, fat on the inside.

Although not part of its current clinical definition, metabolic syndrome has also been linked to non-alcoholic fatty-liver disease, erectile dysfunction in men, polycystic ovarian syndrome (PCOS) in women (a leading cause of infertility and an early indicator of insulin resistance and type 2 diabetes), obstructive sleep apnoea, certain cancers, osteoarthritis, inflammation and increased risk of blood clots.

Numerous studies have demonstrated a link between consumption of added sugar and the onset of metabolic syndrome symptoms. Indeed, according to a 2014 analysis by Quanhe Yang and his colleagues, both epidemiological studies and randomised clinical trials have demonstrated that heavy users of sugar (particularly sugary drinks) tend to be overweight and obese, and are more likely to develop type 2 diabetes, dyslipidemia, cardiovascular disease and high blood pressure. Their own investigation detected a significant relationship between the consumption of added sugars and increased risk of death from cardiovascular disease.

While it's clear that added-sugar consumption is not good for us – as anybody who has witnessed well-behaved children abruptly morph into a crashing, careening conga line of banshees within minutes of consuming a sugar buffet will attest – exactly how sugar harms us is the subject of much debate.

Common table sugar or sucrose is a carbohydrate made up of one molecule of glucose bound to one molecule of fructose. What researchers and stakeholders can't seem to agree on, however, is whether the fructose constituent of sugar is to blame for none, some or all of the problems of which it stands accused. In addition, many studies refer to sucrose, glucose, fructose or high-fructose corn syrup (which contains 55 per cent fructose and 41 per cent glucose) simply as sugar, making it difficult to obtain a common reference point.

Professor Luc Tappy, a prominent obesity and metabolism researcher from the University of Lausanne in Switzerland, notes that fructose does not appear to be required for any known physiological functions, whereas glucose is required by all cells of the body to generate energy. In addition, we do not need to consume sucrose to obtain the glucose we require, as we can acquire it from complex carbohydrates. According to Tappy, sucrose is not only non-essential but is responsible for two problematic consequences: the rapid digestion of sucrose leads to surges in blood glucose that may interfere with insulin; and the fructose component when consumed in high levels places stress on the liver that can lead to increased levels of triglycerides and very low-density lipoprotein (VLDL, which transports triglycerides) in the blood. Circulating VLDL is significantly associated with cardiovascular disease.

In animal experiments, feeding them large amounts of sucrose or fructose results in the development of obesity, insulin resistance, diabetes, dyslipidemia and sometimes high blood pressure, all of which are symptoms of metabolic syndrome and may ultimately lead to cardiovascular disease. In addition, fructose is the only sugar that can elevate uric acid concentrations in the blood, which may result in painful gout or kidney stones.

Critics of the fructose theory of metabolic syndrome generally point to a number of flaws in the overarching argument. First, fructose experiments often involve feeding large amounts of only fructose to animals or people, an unlikely real-life scenario given most people consume sucrose. Secondly, given that large amounts of fructose have been used in studies to achieve an effect, the issue is more about overconsumption than just consumption.

Peripheral nerve damage

In his 2015 book *Sugar Crush: How to Reduce Inflammation, Reverse Nerve Damage, and Reclaim Good Health*, podiatric surgeon Richard Jacoby describes his experience as a young surgical trainee of holding steady the rotting gangrenous leg of a man suffering from diabetic peripheral neuropathy (nerve damage) as it was sawn off just above the knee.

As he struggled with the sound of the saw, the foul stench of the gangrenous leg and the enormous weight of the amputated limb as he carried it to the medical waste bin, little could he have imagined that he would perform thousands of amputations and foot surgeries on rapidly growing numbers of diabetic patients over the next 30 years.

After years of treating patients under the standard model of pharmaceuticals and surgery, Jacoby realised that he was just providing sick care, not health care, and was thus thrilled to become one of the first surgeons to learn the Dellon triple nerve decompression procedure from the inventor himself. This involves reducing pressure on the nerves in the tarsal tunnel (on the inner leg, behind the ankle), restoring blood flow and nerve function to the foot, and dramatically reducing the likelihood of further diabetic ulcers and amputation. When he investigated further why the procedure worked so well, Jacoby came to understand that the compression of the nerves was closely connected to sugar and carbohydrate consumption.

I will leave you to discover the exact mechanics in his book, but Jacoby asserts that sugar flowing constantly through the bloodstream leads to the inflammation and swelling of the nerves to the point that they press against surrounding bone, muscle and tissue. No longer able to send and receive normal nerve impulses, the inflamed nerves generate pain, tingling, burning, itchiness and numbness – the first signs of neuropathy in patients with diabetes or metabolic syndrome.

Jacoby describes the stages of neuropathy, from intermittent pain and numbness in the feet to constant pain and a requirement for painkillers, to finally no pain, just numbness. Then come the ulcers that don't heal, and the amputations. Jacoby asserts that irrespective of the phase you are in or even whether you have received a diagnosis or not, developing neuropathy stems from 'a diet that's full of sugar'.

Dr Jacoby's book makes sober reading for anybody still not convinced about the health risks associated with sugar consumption, and he pulls no punches with his patients: 'the choice is pretty simple: change your diet or lose your foot'. Indeed, his list of allied diseases commonly found in patients with metabolic syndrome would make even the most rigid supporter of the status quo rethink their excessive consumption of sugar and refined carbohydrate.

In an interesting aside, it would appear that sugar can at least offer people with diabetic foot ulcers a cheap alternative to typical wound-healing options. Although the application of sugar to wounds may sound counterintuitive, many studies have shown that 'sugar therapy' can achieve remarkable results. While the mechanisms for its success are not entirely clear, one group of researchers who achieved a 99.2 per cent cure rate in 120 patients with infected wounds concluded that sugar destroys bacteria, draws immune cells to the wound, promotes cleaning of the wound, and reduces local inflammation and swelling. Further studies on diabetic ulcers have demonstrated positive results, although the authors note that larger trials are needed. It's worth noting that sugar has been used for wound healing since Egyptian times, and is still in Latin America, Africa, Europe and Asia, but the practice has not been widespread in English-speaking countries.

Telomere damage

Can sugar harm us in other ways? In a 2014 study, researchers looked at whether there could be a link between sugar-sweetened beverage consumption and the deterioration of telomeres. A telomere is a protective cap that sits over the end of our chromosomes to prevent the arms from eroding. Shortened telomeres are considered to be biomarkers of high oxidative stress, inflammation, chronic life stress, ageing and a shortened life span.

The researchers measured telomeres by obtaining stored DNA from 5309 people aged 20–65 with no history of diabetes or cardiovascular disease. They found that consumption of sugar-sweetened drinks was associated with shortened telomeres, while drinks made from 100 per cent fruit juice were associated with longer telomeres. The researchers also calculated that damage caused to telomeres by daily consumption of a 590-millilitre bottle of sugar-sweetened drink might be comparable to that from smoking. Given that many children and young adults now consume soft drinks on a regular basis, the possibility of telomere damage is worrying.

To make things worse, a 2014 systematic review and meta-analysis of 24 studies involving 24,725 participants demonstrated an inverse association between telomere length and coronary heart disease. A 2005 study also revealed that the telomeres of obese women were significantly shorter than those of lean women, and as we know, obesity is a risk factor for numerous chronic conditions.

Cancer

Cancer appears to be yet another 'disease of civilisation' that was rare among indigenous peoples until the arrival of sugar, refined wheat and seed oil. Indeed, Aboriginal and Torres Strait Islanders, a group for whom malignancy was virtually unheard of, today have a higher incidence of cancer and mortality than non-Indigenous Australians. Moreover, their ability to survive cancer treatment is lower. Indigenous women diagnosed with breast cancer during 2003–07 had a 100 per cent higher risk of dying from any cause by 2010 than non-Indigenous women. In addition, Indigenous women were 2.8 times more likely to develop cervical cancer than non-Indigenous women and 3.9 times more likely to die from it. That Indigenous Australians consume high levels of sugar is well known; some of the highest per-capita soft-drink consumption figures are attributed to the Northern Territory.

According to a 2007 report, *Food, Nutrition, Physical Activity and the Prevention of Cancer: A Global Perspective*, by the World Cancer Research Fund and the American Institute for Cancer Research, the evidence that obesity is involved in colorectal, oesophageal, endometrial, pancreatic, kidney and, after menopause, breast cancer is convincing. According to the report, insulin resistance is more common among obese people, leading to high levels of insulin in the blood, which increases the risk of colon and endometrial cancers, and potentially of pancreatic and kidney cancer as well. Increased circulating leptin levels are also associated with colorectal and prostate cancers in obese people. And finally, elevated levels of sex steroid hormones such as oestrogens, androgens (such as testosterone) and progesterone are often found in obese people and are strongly associated with an increased risk of endometrial and postmenopausal breast cancers.

The World Cancer Research Fund notes maintaining weight in the healthy range and avoidance of alcohol and sugary drinks as being some of the best ways to reduce your risk of developing the most common cancers.

Pro and anti-cancer effects of weight, nutrition, PUFA and physical activity

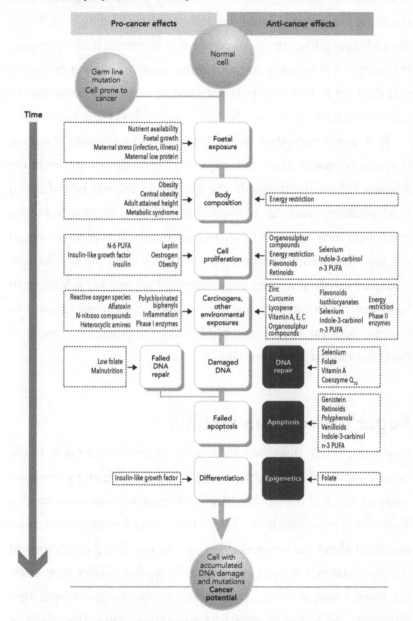

Adapted from: American Institute for Cancer Research
(PUFA stands for Polyunsaturated fatty acids)

Intestinal permeability

In the normal human gut, a small amount of material passes from inside the gut into the rest of the body via the gut lining cells. While this cell layer allows the passage of some nutrients, it also prevents the escape of potentially harmful substances. It has been proposed that damage to this barrier is involved in numerous autoimmune conditions, leading to a condition known as leaky gut syndrome.

In a paper published in the journal *Autoimmunity Reviews*, researchers noted that the explosive growth in autoimmune diseases fell neatly alongside the growth in the use of industrial food additives such as nanoparticles, gluten, organic solvents, emulsifiers such as soy lecithin, and sugars. Because glucose is used not just as a flavour enhancer but also as an absorption enhancer, it may be involved in increasing intestinal permeability, leading to leaky gut syndrome. In laboratory studies, glucose was shown to increase permeability of cultured human cells used as a model of the intestinal barrier in humans.

Sugar's forgotten victims

One final, rarely discussed issue with sugar consumption is the living conditions and health of the people growing and processing sugar on much of the world's behalf. (Almost all sugar consumed in Australia is produced here.) Given that many British people, once informed about the unspeakable working and living conditions of the sugar slaves, refused to consume the stuff; and once they knew the truth about slavery, created the abolitionist movement that ultimately led to the world's first anti-slavery laws, the plight of those still living and working in the world's sugar-cane fields and processing plants must not go unmentioned when exploring the subject of sugar and health.

Over the last twenty years, poverty-stricken Central American sugar-cane workers from El Salvador, Nicaragua, Costa Rica, Guatemala, Panama, Honduras and southern Mexico have fallen victim in their tens of thousands to a type of kidney failure usefully called chronic kidney disease of unknown origin (CKDu).

In the Nicaraguan municipality of Chichigalpa, home to Ingenio San Antonio (ISA) the country's oldest and largest sugar mill, CKDu has been responsible for almost half the male deaths recorded in the last ten years. So many of fathers, sons, brothers and uncles have succumbed to the disease in Chichigalpa that it's now known as La Isla du Viudas or the Island of Widows. Seven out of ten men there now have CKDu, and the disease has also become the leading cause of male adult deaths in hospitals in El Salvador.

CKDu is different from chronic kidney disease (CKD), which mainly affects wealthy nations and is mostly caused by obesity, high blood pressure and type 2 diabetes – in other words, metabolic syndrome. While researchers have debated the exact cause of CKDu, it's believed to be a combination of heat and dehydration, exposure to agricultural chemicals and consumption of hard water. Indeed, many workers struck down with the condition have been known to routinely work excessive shifts, cutting sugar cane with a machete in oppressive heat, with little or no water available for hydration. Cutting sugar cane manually is known to be one of the most backbreaking jobs in the world. In addition, agricultural chemicals are widely used and workers do not have access to protective clothing.

Nicaragua is the second-poorest country in the Americas after Haiti, and the ISA plantation, owned by 'the sugar king' and Nicaragua's first billionaire, Carlos Pellas, is considered ground zero in the battle for changes to work conditions, and for access to company-held medical records, ongoing medical care and compensation. While CKDu is officially recognised as a possible work-related illness, to qualify for benefits and specialist health care, workers must prove they became sick while working. Workers say, however, that ISA will not provide sick workers with a copy of their medical records.

Workers undergo medical tests at the beginning of each harvest and are refused further work once their tests reveal kidney damage.

'I was healthy when I started working for the company and sick when they got rid of me,' said one worker. 'Every family here has lost someone, the work is making us sick, but there are no alternatives. We are all dying from it, it's a total epidemic.'

ISA refuses to accept liability, noting that scientific studies have been unable to determine the causes of CKDu or establish a causal link between sugar-cane work and the disease, basing its statement on a review of scientific literature carried out by Boston University and paid for by . . . ISA. In a further attempt to distance its work practices from the illness, ISA and the Nicaraguan sugar-cane industry are now funding Boston University to conduct further research that aims to understand genetic and childhood links to the disease. Like most industry-sponsored 'research' the findings will no doubt 'deepen the mystery' and 'raise more questions than answers', thus enabling ISA and companies like it to ignore their negative externalities. Such smokescreens may maintain the status quo for companies doing the wrong thing, but as always will accomplish nothing for the suffering workers, who will continue to take part in the harvest and give their lives for the world's next sugar hit.

In December 2014, a group of sick cane cutters and widows walked 130 kilometres in scorching heat to Nicaragua's capital, Managua, hoping to take their case to government representatives.

One protester stated, 'Whole families are being wiped out by this illness, we want to be compensated fairly, and make sure every sick worker has access to medical treatment, this is our right.' The government of President José Ortega, which is known to have close ties to Carlos Pellas, did not respond to the marchers.

It's apparent that Western Price's indigenous research subjects and Western consumers are not and never have been the sole victims of sugar's deadly spread throughout our food supply. From the millions of Africans taken from their homes and forced to work the sugar plantations of old, to the poverty-stricken and desperately sick Central American farmers of today, our sugar addiction has come at enormous cost to the communities and individuals our favourite sweeter has touched.

What we need to ask ourselves is whether suffering, destruction and death are really the price we want to pay for 'the sweet stuff'.

7

Can wheat make us sick?

In 1979 *Washington Post* investigative journalist Dan Morgan published his bestselling book titled *The Merchants of Grain: The Power and Profits of the Five Giant Companies at the Centre of the World's Food Supply*. The book is widely considered to be the closest a journalist has yet come to exposing the machinations of the global grain supply and the secretive families that have traditionally controlled the market.

While the book is worth reading if you want to develop an understanding of how commodity markets work, a chapter titled 'Cram it down their throats' is perhaps the most illuminating in terms of describing the mindset of those who are more than happy to witness their grain cement itself as the foundation of not just the Western diet but the carbohydrate-heavy food pyramid. If you have ever wondered why the USDA advised US citizens to consume an excessive six to eleven servings of carbohydrate-heavy grain per day, the book may offer a number of insights.

The indigenous groups Weston Price studied found out the hard way that including refined-wheat products in their diet had deleterious effects. Not one of these groups consumed refined wheat before the arrival of European traders, and yet the consequences of them doing so became quickly and painfully apparent. While Price asserted that it was the processing or demineralising of wheat that caused the problem, an abundance of recent scientific evidence has provided significant insight into several mechanisms by which consumption of wheat (refined or not) might negatively affect our health.

The trouble with gluten

Gluten avoidance has been a hot topic for several years now, with everyone from Gwyneth Paltrow to Bill and Chelsea Clinton, Victoria Beckham, Miley Cyrus, Russell Crowe, Novak Djokovic and Rachel Weisz now openly avoiding gluten-containing foods. A June 2013 consumer survey conducted in the United States by market research company Mintel revealed that of the consumers questioned who were eating gluten-free foods, 36 per cent were doing so for reasons other than sensitivity or intolerance, 28 per cent had been diagnosed with coeliac disease by a doctor; a further 28 per cent had not been diagnosed by a doctor but suffered from gluten-intolerance symptoms such as abdominal pain, indigestion, foggy mind, fatigue or headaches upon consumption; and 9 per cent were avoiding gluten to see if it really was causing a problem for them. Billions of dollars are now spent globally on gluten-free foods, so what is gluten and why might we benefit from removing it from our diet?

WHAT IS GLUTEN?

A grain of wheat consists of three parts:

1. the bran, the outer shell of the kernel, which provides vitamins, minerals and fibre
2. the germ, the plant embryo, which provides antioxidants and vitamins
3. the endosperm, comprising more than 80 per cent of the grain, which provides protein and carbohydrate.

The endosperm is the fuel store of the grain and contains the starchy component and gluten. Gluten (Latin for 'glue') is the major structural protein of wheat. It consists of a group of prolamins (storage proteins) called glutenins and gliadins. It's these glutenins and gliadins that, when mixed with water, give the wheat the visco-elasticity vital for making bread, pastries, pasta and other foods. It also helps dough to rise and retains moisture, enabling breads and buns to stay fresher for longer.

Coeliac disease

Gluten is most closely associated with coeliac disease (CD), a once-rare condition that today affects around one in 100 people. The prevalence of CD is rapidly growing in a manner inconsistent with better detection rates, and has increasingly been put down to changes in wheat-breeding practices. CD occurs when the body treats gluten as a foreign invader and mounts an immune response against it. This occurs mainly in the small intestine and is treated by excluding gluten from the diet. Symptoms can be gastrointestinal, including bloating, abdominal pain and distension, gas, weight loss, diarrhoea and fatty stools. Non-gastrointestinal symptoms are many and varied, and include skin disorders, anaemia, joint pains, bone disorders and headaches. If left untreated, CD can lead to more serious diseases such as lymphoma, infertility, osteoporosis, cancer and death. There is a strong genetic component that predisposes some people to developing CD, but it can strike anyone at any stage of their life.

Dermatitis herpetiformis

Another gluten-related condition, which shares a proven link with CD, is dermatitis herpetiformis (DH). DH appears as a blistering rash that when scratched results in broken skin and scarring. It's most often found around the elbows, knees and shoulders, and sufferers experience itching and burning sensations before an outbreak of papules or blisters.

Researchers have noted that a number of genes coding for an immune response and inflammation are up-regulated or over-expressed in DH. In addition, genes that code for apoptosis (cell destruction), cell proliferation and extracellular matrix (wound repair) were also up-regulated. Genes for proteins at the dermal–epidermal junction (where blister formation occurs) and metabolism were mostly down-regulated or under-expressed. In all, the researchers found 72 differentially expressed genes involved in the development of skin lesions in DH, a disease triggered by gluten consumption.

Wheat allergy

Wheat allergy includes four main conditions. These are:

1. **respiratory allergy,** also known as 'baker's cough' or 'baker's asthma' which affects 4.2 per cent of bakery workers in their first year, rising to 8.6 per cent in their second year, and includes symptoms such as wheezing, itching and coughing
2. **food allergy,** which can involve the gastrointestinal tract, skin and/or respiratory tract
3. **wheat-dependent, exercise-induced anaphylaxis,** which occurs either during or immediately after exercise when wheat is consumed
4. **contact urticaria,** a blistering rash.

Non-coeliac gluten sensitivity

In addition to coeliac disease, gluten appears to play a role in a newly described condition called non-coeliac gluten sensitivity (NCGS). NCGS differs from coeliac disease in that it has so far not been proven to have a strong heredity basis, a connection to poor absorption of gluten, nutritional deficiencies, or an increased risk of autoimmune issues or cancer.

Researchers first raised the possibility of NCGS in 1980, when they discovered that some people devoid of the CD diagnostic criteria, yet clearly suffering from gastrointestinal problems such as diarrhoea and bloating, were relieved of their symptoms on a gluten-free diet. In recent years, increasing numbers of people have reported a range of symptoms that have been ameliorated via a gluten-free diet. These symptoms include gastrointestinal problems such as bloating, constipation, nausea, reflux, abdominal pain, diarrhoea, and systemic symptoms such as skin rashes, headache, depression, brain fog, anxiety, fatigue, fibromyalgia-type muscle and joint pain, arm or leg numbness, dermatitis and anaemia. Pasquale Mansueto and his colleagues pointed out that people suffering from NCGS (once CD, DH, gluten ataxia [see page 183] or wheat allergy have been excluded) show wide variation in the genesis and development of their symptoms.

In recent times, experts have proposed that the term non-coeliac gluten sensitivity might be replaced with the term non-coeliac wheat sensitivity. In addition to the understanding that some people may be FODMAP sensitive (see page 183) has come a realisation that other aspects or fragments of wheat apart from gluten might be driving consumer claims of gluten intolerance and the increased demand for gluten-free diets and foods.

Far more research is required to determine the true nature and prevalence of NCGS, including clear and accurate definitions of its subgroups, such as FODMAP sensitivity. Ideally, accurate, reliable biomarkers for NCGS will be established, along with simple and inexpensive testing methods, to enable consumers to know where they stand. Many people I interviewed for this book, including those who successfully resolved their depression by following a gluten-free diet, spoke of their distress at reporting NCGS symptoms to their doctor and being ridiculed as result. This is unacceptable given the condition is recognised by leading experts in the field and listed in the 'Oslo definitions for coeliac disease and related terms' published in 2013. 'Diagnosis of non-coeliac gluten sensitivity (NCGS): the Salerno Experts Criteria', published June 2015, includes a diagnostic evaluation procedure for doctors and NCGS patients in the absence of 'sensitive and specific biomarkers'.

Gluten, zonulin and intestinal permeability

As noted earlier, gluten contains prolamins, which consist of glutenins and gliadins. Gliadin is the component most associated with the development of coeliac disease in those with a genetic predisposition. Gliadin has been shown to increase intestinal permeability via its ability to up-regulate the protein zonulin, which directly compromises the barrier function of the gut. Once this occurs, these 'leaks' permit dietary and microbial antigens to enter the bloodstream and begin interacting with cells of the immune system throughout the body.

In his August 2009 article 'Surprises from celiac disease', featured in *Scientific American*, Professor Alessio Fasano described his team's accidental discovery of the protein zonulin. In the late 1980s, they were trying, unsuccessfully, to develop a vaccine for cholera when they discovered a toxin that could induce the tight junctions between adjacent cells to 'leak'. This was eventually identified as zonulin, a protein secreted by cells lining the intestines as well as cells found in other tissues and organs. Zonulin has been found to increase intestinal permeability and regulates 'the movement of fluid, large molecules and immune cells between body compartments'. Fasano is famous for his maxim: 'The gut is not like Las Vegas. What happens in the gut does not stay in the gut.' In other words, intestinal permeability can cause serious problems in tissues and organs located far from the main trouble spot, the gut.

In the article, Fasano notes that the discovery of zonulin prompted his team to search the medical literature for other health disorders that involved intestinal permeability. This resulted in the surprising revelation that numerous autoimmune diseases, including coeliac disease, type 1 diabetes, multiple sclerosis, rheumatoid arthritis and inflammatory bowel disease, feature problems with intestinal permeability. It has since been shown that, in several of these diseases, intestinal permeability is caused by unusually high levels of zonulin, and research into coeliac disease has demonstrated that gliadin in wheat causes increased secretion of zonulin.

In March 2015, many years after the discovery of zonulin, a research paper was published that sought to answer an important question regarding intestinal permeability. Does wheat gliadin cause the up-regulation of zonulin only in people with coeliac disease or in everybody? The research group took biopsies from the duodenum (first part of the small intestine after the stomach) in four groups, including:

1. coeliac patients with active disease
2. coeliac patients in remission
3. non-coeliac patients with gluten sensitivity
4. non-coeliac controls.

The samples were incubated with gliadin or neutral media. The tissues from all groups demonstrated an increase in permeability when exposed to gliadin, and those from patients with gluten sensitivity or active coeliac disease demonstrated greater levels of intestinal permeability than those of coeliac disease patients who were in remission. This study concluded that gliadin was capable of inducing intestinal permeability in all individuals, irrespective of any underlying condition.

In his many interviews and presentations, Fasano stresses that while CD is the only specific autoimmune disease where a precise environmental trigger (gluten) has been positively identified, it provides valuable clues to the autoimmune process and directions for future research and therapies. In addition, Fasano has often pointed to a growing body of evidence suggesting a number of factors involved in the development of autoimmune disease: an environmental substance; a genetic predisposition; and intestinal permeability. Such an understanding, Fasano asserts, suggests that removing one 'leg of the autoimmune stool' should theoretically be enough to stop the disease process.

It's worth noting that in recent years, and with more research under his belt, Fasano added two further components to his auto-immune disease recipe: an imbalanced gut microbiota; and an inappropriate response of the innate immune system.

Gluten and the brain

Gluten can also be a problem for the brain. In 2013, neurologist Marios Hadjivassiliou and gastroenterologist David Sanders established the Sheffield Institute of Gluten-Related Disorders, the first clinic in the world to focus on the neurological manifestations of gluten consumption. Professor Hadjivassiliou first realised a connection between patients with balance and movement problems and the presence of anti-gliadin antibodies (AGA) in the 1990s.

Much of his work has centred on understanding the extent to which gluten can affect the brain. His work in the area of these movement problems, now known as gluten ataxia (GA), revealed that more than half of patients diagnosed with the condition do not have gastrointestinal symptoms, indicating that for those people gluten toxicity is manifested in the brain and nervous system. Hadjivassiliou's open mind and lateral thinking enabled him to notice the connections between seemingly disparate symptoms such as peripheral nerve damage and headaches, and the presence of gluten-related antibodies. He also noticed the resolution of a broad range of symptoms on the gluten free-diet, which he prescribes as part of his GA treatment.

Professor Fasano writes in his 2014 book *Gluten Freedom: The Nation's Leading Expert Offers the Essential Guide to a Healthy, Gluten-Free Lifestyle* about some of the research undertaken in the field of gluten and brain disorders, including schizophrenia and autism spectrum disorders.

The link between gluten and schizophrenia was first noted in the 1966 paper 'Wheat consumption and hospital admissions for schizophrenia during World War II', which found that admissions to mental hospitals for schizophrenia fell during some wars, possibly due to severely diminished supplies of gluten-containing grains. Also noted was the fact that emotional disturbances were usually the first symptoms to dissipate in coeliac disease patients upon commencement of a gluten-free diet. In addition, a 2006 literature review on the subject found that in many cases a drastic reduction or full remission of schizophrenic symptoms could be achieved via a gluten-free diet.

A 1984 study found only two chronic schizophrenics among more than 65,000 examined or observed adults in remote parts of Papua New Guinea, the Solomon Islands and Yap in Micronesia, where grains weren't consumed. The researchers noted that when these people consumed wheat, barley and rice, the prevalence of schizophrenia reached European levels.

A 2015 paper titled 'Gluten psychosis: confirmation of a new clinical entity' described the case of a fourteen-year-old girl who suffered from the onset of severe hallucinations and psychotic behaviour. After repeated admissions to a psychiatric ward and numerous diagnostic tests, she was prescribed a gluten-free diet for seemingly separate gastrointestinal problems not related to coeliac disease. Within days, the symptoms of her psychiatric condition diminished before vanishing altogether. The child was able to drop her medications, and nine months after adopting the gluten-free diet she was still symptom-free and, according to her mother, 'a normal girl'. The paper reports that even accidental ingestion of minute levels of gluten could, within four hours, trigger psychotic symptoms from which it took the girl three days to recover fully. While this is not to say that all mental illness is related to gluten ingestion, it does suggest that dietary issues may play a role for some people.

Other components of wheat

Some people who follow a gluten-free diet actually experience improvements in their system due to the removal not of gluten but of other components in wheat that can cause a variety of health problems.

FODMAP sensitivity

Recent studies have suggested that claims of gluten sensitivity may actually be cases of FODMAP sensitivity. These studies, however, appear to address only the gastrointestinal aspects of the non-CD gluten problem and have failed to provide an explanation for the systemic symptoms such as joint pains, depression, skin conditions and autoimmunity.

Omega-6 in wheat

As discussed in Chapter 5, excessive linoleic acid or omega-6 in the diet is understood to be involved in a broad range of health conditions, but seed oils are not the only food with high levels of linoleic acid. According to the USDA, 1 US cup (142 grams) of white wheat flour contains:

- 0.5 grams of saturated fat
- 0.4 grams of monounsaturated fat
- 1.4 grams of polyunsaturated fat, of which:
  - 67.2 milligrams is total omega-3
  - 1.373 grams is total omega-6.

One cup of wholegrain flour is not much better, with:

- 45.6 milligrams of omega-3, and
- 886 milligrams of omega-6.

While these figures are nowhere near the omega-6 content of seed oil, it's easy to see how frequent consumption of wheat may contribute to the overload of omega-6 in the average diet, and may also contribute to the many diseases associated with AA cascade overreactions (see page 128) and a flooded endocannabinoid system (see page 138). Researchers have noted that both anandamide and cannabinoid receptors are found in the gastrointestinal tract, and a dysregulated system is understood to play a role in diseases of the gut including diarrhoea, colon cancer, coeliac disease and inflammatory and irritable bowel disease. Indeed, studies suggest a dysregulated endocannabinoid system may play a role in the development of coeliac disease. Could aspects of non-coeliac gluten intolerance, such as brain fog, depression, fatigue, osteoporosis, joint problems and weight problems, actually be explained by this connection?

Lipopolysaccharides

Lipopolysaccharides, also known as endotoxins, are cell-wall fragments from some of the bacteria that reside for the most part in our gut. Lipopolysaccharides are known to be involved in chronic inflammation due to their ability to bind to receptors on our cells that activate an immune response.

While endotoxins can evidently be found in low amounts in a normal person's circulation, they are commonly found in increased levels in the bloodstream of those with metabolic syndrome; non-alcoholic fatty-liver disease; cardiovascular diseases; inflammatory bowel diseases; and neurological and psychiatric diseases including autism, Lou Gehrig's disease, Parkinson's and Alzheimer's. This has led to greater interest in the issue of endotoxemia – high levels of endotoxins in the blood. Elevated blood levels of major defence antibodies directed against lipopolysaccharides have also been implicated in major depression and chronic fatigue syndrome.

While higher endotoxin levels in the blood have been related to chronic stress, heat stress, junk-food diets and alcohol consumption, it's possible that the zonulin-inducing aspect of gluten-containing grains in also involved. One study conducted in India revealed that blood levels of lipopolysaccharides and human-produced zonulin were significantly increased in type 2 diabetics. This implies that in places (unlike India) where wheat is a staple, lipopolysaccharide levels may be even more elevated.

Studies have also shown connections between lipopolysaccharides, dietary fats and the AA cascade. In one of these, mice were injected with lipopolysaccharide from E. *coli* and then fed a low-fat diet or diets high in fish oil, safflower oil, coconut oil or olive oil. The mice on the fish oil and coconut oil diets showed lower levels of inflammatory markers, while those markers were highest in mice fed the low-fat and safflower oil diets. The authors expressed alarm at this situation, because formulas for intravenous feeding given to patients with infectious diseases are based on omega-6 soybean oil, which could lead to an over-production of pro-inflammatory immune-signalling compounds (cytokines), resulting in immune system dysfunction, septic shock and multiple organ failure.

Wheat amylase trypsin inhibitors

Wheat amylase trypsin inhibitors (ATIs) are a family of seventeen wheat proteins that make up around 4 per cent of total wheat protein and are increasingly believed to play a role in NCGS. Wheat ATIs can activate the same immune-signalling receptors as endotoxins and create an inflammatory intestinal response. They are also understood to play a role in other immune-related diseases, both inside and outside the gastrointestinal tract, such as baker's asthma, in which they are believed to be the key allergen.

The ATI content of wheat has drastically increased over recent years due to breeding of high-yield, highly pest-resistant wheat, and ATIs are considered to be part of the plant's pest-resistance mechanism.

Lectins and wheatgerm agglutinin

Wheatgerm agglutinin (WGA) is a lectin specific to the wheat plant. Lectins (from the Latin *legere*, meaning 'to select') are defined as non-immune carbohydrate-binding proteins that can specifically recognise and reversibly bind to carbohydrates without altering their structure. This means that lectins have the unique ability to stick to carbohydrates on the surface of our individual cells, but can unstick if they detect a preferred sugar group.

Autoimmunity, cancer and cancer metastases are understood to have links to both lectins and aberrant linkage of sugars to other compounds. Indeed, according to one research group, 'plant lectins (e.g. wheatgerm agglutinin) showed enhanced binding to and agglutination of tumor cells'. WGA has also been linked to type 1 and type 2 diabetes.

The role that lectins play within a plant is in some cases not well understood, but what is known is that lectins can act as a defence protein. Their role as internal plant pesticide is to deter predators (including us) from consuming the seed that ensures the future of the species. Not all plant lectins are considered toxic to humans, and most are excreted by the human digestive tract, but evidence suggests that apart from WGA, agglutinins from soybeans, peanuts and kidney beans can negatively influence human cells.

According to Arpad Pusztai, a Hungarian-born biochemist and nutritionist called the 'father of lectinology', some food allergies might actually be immune system responses to the presence of lectins. After a decades-long career studying lectins, in 1993 he raised the issue of WGA and its potential to harm animals.

In 1999, the eminent allergist and immunologist David L. J. Freed directly posed the question 'Do dietary lectins cause disease?', suggesting that sufficient evidence was available to underpin a discussion. Freed noted that wheat consumption has been linked to rheumatoid arthritis (an issue explored further by Loren Cordain, the 'father of Paleo'). Anecdotally, sufferers of rheumatoid arthritis have been known to 'live' on glucosamine tablets in an effort to experience relief, and this may be due to the fact that antibodies in rheumatoid disease terminate not in the usual galactose but in N-acetyl glucosamine, to which WGA specifically binds. It comes as no surprise, then, that sufferers of rheumatoid arthritis feel better on a wheat-free diet.

Many dogs today also experience crippling arthritis, and some pet-food brands now contain added glucosamine. Glucosamine tablets for dogs are also strong sellers in pet-food stores. Given processed wheat is a relatively new addition to the diet of dogs (in processed dog crunches, biscuits and canned foods), could it be possible that WGA is entering their system and harming their joints and possibly other tissues? Several of the high-end dog foods have become 'gluten-free', so perhaps the industry has started to capitalise on this growing problem. Although dogs are omnivores, processed-wheat consumption is highly unnatural for them, so perhaps a gluten-free diet is the best option in any case, but particularly for breeds with a high level of susceptibility to arthritis.

Possibly the best known diet that deals specifically with dietary lectins is the 'blood-type' diet made famous by Peter D'Adamo. Inspired by the phrase 'one man's meat is another man's poison',

D'Adamo's father, James, also a doctor, sought to understand why some people lost weight on a certain diet while others gained it; why dairy products produced mucus in some people but not others; and why high-protein diets seemed optimal for some but less than optimal for others. James D'Adamo concluded that our blood type may play a role in our health based on how our blood reacts to lectins. The blood-type diet forbids gluten-containing grains and legumes for type O blood (the most common blood type, said to have evolved in our hunter-gatherer ancestors) due to their lectin content.

Researchers from the University of Toronto published a 'debunking' study of the blood-type diet in 2014. They assessed the dietary intake of 1455 people using a one-month, 196-item food-frequency questionnaire that applied a score to determine relative adherence to each of the four blood-type diets. One major issue concerning this questionnaire was that it included processed and junk foods such as pizza, French fries and hamburgers, none of which is included in the D'Adamo diet. Furthermore, it listed sandwiches, hotdogs and hamburgers with wheat bread as suitable foods for people with type O blood, but the blood-type diet restricts wheat for these people due to the effects of WGA on their system.

While a 2014 article in the *Journal of Cereal Science* asserted that there have been no randomised controlled trials in humans regarding the effect of WGA consumption, numerous researchers have found evidence that WGA can play a role in inflammation, intestinal permeability and altered immune response in humans.

Anti-nutrient properties

Wheat contains phytic acid (also known as phytate), which is the storage form of phosphorus and a demineraliser of the vital minerals iron, zinc, calcium and magnesium. This demineralising effect becomes a problem when a large portion of an individual's diet consists of wheat-based products such as bread, cereals and pasta, as the minerals are carried out of our bodies rather than delivered to our cells where they are needed.

Iron

Iron deficiency is the most common mineral deficiency in the world, and an estimated 1.6 billion people or a quarter of the world's population are suffering from iron-deficiency anaemia. Iron is a vital part of the blood's oxygen-carrying molecule haemoglobin, each one of which carries up to four oxygen atoms. Iron is also needed for more than 90 enzymes, including those involved in producing the energy molecules used by our cells as well as testosterone and oestrogen, and an enzyme that kills bacteria, myeloperoxidase. Iron is also required for the transport of fatty acids to cells to make energy, and the synthesis of serotonin (to prevent depression) and adrenaline.

Even before I developed kidney disease, I always grappled with maintaining my iron levels, and the problem became much worse once I was a dialysis patient. I struggled to find a supplement that worked, and the brands prescribed by doctors didn't really agree with my system. When I was released from hospital after my transplant, I had a haemoglobin level of 6 grams per decilitre, which is very low (low is defined as less than 12 grams per decilitre for women and less than 13.5 grams per decilitre for men). Once life began to normalise, I decided to remove gluten from my diet and started to take a particular brand of iron. This seemed to do the trick, and my haemoglobin levels shot up very quickly to 13 grams per decilitre. Even today I have to keep up the supplementation, but I sometimes wonder if my previous gluten-heavy diet was hindering my ability to absorb enough iron.

Calcium

Calcium plays an essential role in activating the secretion of hormones, including insulin and calcitonin (which helps maintain calcium levels in the blood), and helps lower blood pressure and cholesterol levels. It regulates our heartbeat and is involved in muscle contraction, nerve impulse transmission and blood clotting. It's also involved in bone and tooth formation. Vitamins A, C, D and K and phosphorus must also be available for calcium to work properly in the body. Some of the highest dietary sources of calcium include dairy products, almonds, broccoli, green leafy vegetables and bone soup.

According to a nutrition survey conducted in the United States, overweight people and those with a low income were at greater risk of calcium and vitamin D deficiency, while large numbers of the US population likely did not obtain sufficient calcium from diet alone. Too much calcium (known as hypercalcemia) can cause many health problems as well, so it's important to know your status before taking a supplement.

Magnesium

The milling of wheat results in a loss of around 90 per cent of its magnesium, making refined wheat a poor source of this mineral. In addition, phytates in wheat bind to magnesium and remove it from the body. A balance of magnesium and calcium is vital for proper nerve function, but when magnesium deficiency occurs, a build-up of calcium can result. Magnesium deficiency potentially affects around half the population, which is of particular concern given long-term deficiency has been linked with insulin resistance, high blood glucose, calcium build-up in tissues and joints, and kidney and gallstones.

Magnesium is important for around 300 enzymes in the body and is required for the activation of numerous vitamins, including vitamin D, and minerals. It's involved in the production of the molecule cells use for energy and of serotonin, maintenance of heart muscle and relaxation of blood vessels. It regulates body temperature and plays a role in fat metabolism. Too much magnesium can also cause health problems, so your levels should be determined before you increase your intake.

Zinc

US professor of biochemistry and molecular biochemistry Bruce Ames, one of America's best known scientists, created the Ames test, a cheap way to test for potential carcinogens in consumer products. He showed that cigarette smoke can cause DNA mutations, but he is also one of the world's experts on micronutrients. He was involved, for example, in the discovery that iron deficiency causes neuron (nerve cell) decay and damage to mitochondrial DNA, while folate deficiency breaks chromosomes in a similar fashion to radiation.

Ames also knows a lot about zinc, another vital mineral bound and removed from the body by phytate in cereal grains such as wheat and in legumes. Zinc is required for more than 1000 proteins in the body, including some involved in repairing damaged DNA. Ames's research suggests that a combination of low zinc intake and high phytate intake can reduce the ability to handle oxidative stress and DNA repair, resulting in disease susceptibility.

Zinc deficiency in children can lead to stunted growth, learning difficulties, behavioural problems and poor motor skills. It can also cause diarrhoea in malnourished children and is thought to play a major role in infant and early childhood deaths. Zinc is extremely important for male and female reproductive function and prenatal development, which may be why we associate oysters, which are very high in zinc, with virility. Zinc deficiency is associated with birth defects, weight loss, reduced testosterone in males, auto-immunity, high blood pressure, repeat infections, delayed wound healing, acne, allergies and asthma. Anecdotally, people who take regular zinc supplements also report diminished sugar cravings.

It's worth noting that while all grains, seeds, nuts and legumes contain phytates in varying amounts, this can be affected by how the food is prepared. But problems only arise with heavy, chronic consumption of wheat over months or years.

For the record, Professor Ames asserts that prevention of degenerative diseases will not come from new drugs but healthy metabolism and nutrient density. While Ames admits to a lack of daily exercise, he follows a Mediterranean diet and is still presenting lectures and working in medical research at the age of 88.

Selective breeding of wheat

One of the best known books regarding wheat, heart disease and metabolic syndrome, *Wheat Belly*, was written by American cardiologist William Davis, who managed to stop his own downward health spiral from obesity to type 2 diabetes by removing wheat from his diet. In this book, Davis highlights the fact that our overconsumption of carbohydrates is leading to insulin resistance and the notorious 'wheat belly' common to grain-fed and grain-finished ruminants such as cattle. Davis also controversially claimed that the modern wheat varieties of *Triticum aestivum* used to make most of our processed foods were so radically altered by a US wheat improvement program (funded by the Rockefeller Foundation and the Mexican government) in the early 1940s as to render it downright toxic. Davis put many of his patients on a low-carbohydrate, gluten-free diet and watched as their symptoms of metabolic syndrome, including prediabetes and type 2 diabetes, disappeared.

While some in the scientific community ridiculed Davis for suggesting that selective breeding, which has been going on for thousands of years, could suddenly in the last 50 years cause harm, studies are now starting to emerge that may force a rethink. One 2015 study, a randomised double-blind crossover trial of people with acute coronary syndrome, was designed to test the theory that modern wheat has a different effect on the body from organic ancient wheat, in this instance Khorasan wheat (*Triticum turgidum* subsp. *turicanum*). For the record, the research was funded by the producers of a brand of Khorasan wheat.

The patients were assigned to consume products made either from organic semi-whole Khorasan wheat or, as a control, a mixture of modern organic semi-whole *Triticum aestivum* and *Triticum durum*. The group that consumed the Khorasan products demonstrated lowered total cholesterol, LDL (bad) cholesterol, glucose and insulin 'irrespective of age, sex, traditional risk factors, medication and diet quality'. In addition, there was a significant reduction in molecules that can cause oxidative stress and inflammation. It should also be noted that Khorasan wheat contains higher levels of vanadium than standard modern wheat. Vanadium is a mineral long known to help normalise blood sugar and blood pressure.

In a previous study conducted by the same researchers, a healthy population with no prior clinical symptoms of cardio-vascular disease were placed on a diet using wheat products made with organic Khorasan rather than modern wheat. The diet demonstrated a beneficial effect on cardiovascular risk markers such as total cholesterol, LDL cholesterol, blood glucose, total antioxidant capacity and pro-inflammatory signalling molecules (cytokines). No such effects were observed from a replacement diet using organic, modern wheat products.

A 2014 double-blind, randomised dietary intervention trial revealed that ancient grains had a less damaging effect on patients with irritable bowel syndrome. Symptoms such as abdominal pain, bloating and fatigue lessened, while blood tests demonstrated decreased levels of pro-inflammatory cytokines.

While each of these studies had its limitations, mostly concerning the small numbers of participants and their funding, they lend weight to the claims by William Davis that modern wheat may be contributing to a range of chronic health conditions in susceptible people.

Dietary carbohydrate and metabolic syndrome

When we think of dietary carbohydrates we usually think of wheat-based products such as pasta, bread and bagels, and we might imagine a fit and active athlete 'carbo-loading' before a big race. In reality, however, carbohydrate is just another word for sugars and molecules that combine sugars. As we have seen, the carbohydrate we are most familiar with – table sugar or sucrose – is a disaccharide made up of glucose and fructose. When many sugars combine, they form polysaccharides, such as starch. We know starches as a major component of the refined wheat products most Westerners consume regularly, such as breakfast cereals, bread, pizza, pasta, pies, biscuits and muffins. These may look different from the cans of 'sugar-sweetened beverage' cited by obesity researchers as major culprits in disease, but they are still effectively sugars, and overconsumption contributes to obesity and its many inherent health problems.

Many critics of sugar lay the blame for the explosion of metabolic syndrome and type 2 diabetes at the door of either sugar or its evil constituent fructose. But other researchers disagree that sucrose or fructose is the only culprit, and implicate refined carbohydrates, or carbohydrates generally, as the second half of a somewhat dastardly duo.

A new wave of research

Well-known American biochemist and professor of cell biology Richard Feinman states:

Diabetes is a disease of carbohydrate intolerance. Type 1 is characterised by an inability to produce insulin (a hormone and master controller of the metabolism) in response to carbohydrate. In type 2 there is a peripheral insulin resistance along with deterioration of the [beta] cells of the pancreas. The most salient symptom (and a major contributor to the pathology) is high blood glucose which, not surprisingly, is most effectively treated by reducing dietary carbohydrates ... It is not hard to guess the best treatment for a disease where the defect is a poor response to ingested carbohydrates.

Professor Feinman is among a new wave of scientists and medical researchers currently producing the research that demonstrates the dangerous consequences of the high-carbohydrate, low-fat (high-sugar) diet that has been sold to us by various vested interests and gatekeeping organisations over several decades.

Of particular interest to the low-carbohydrate researchers is the fact that several markers of cardiovascular disease, metabolic syndrome and type 2 diabetes are often eliminated upon the move to a low-carbohydrate diet, and those with these conditions need no drugs to manage them. Indeed, a review published in 2015 noted the abject failure of current dietary recommendations (promoting high carbohydrate and low fat intake) to halt the explosion of type 2 diabetes in any way or even remotely improve obesity, cardiovascular disease or health in general. The authors (26 medical specialists and researchers) state: 'Carbohydrate restriction is the single most effective intervention for reducing all of the features of metabolic syndrome.' They present twelve points of evidence supporting the use of the low-carbohydrate diet as the first approach to type 2 diabetes and as an adjunct to medication in type 1 diabetes:

1. Hyperglycaemia (high blood glucose) is the most salient feature of diabetes. Dietary carbohydrate restriction has the greatest effect on decreasing blood-glucose levels.
2. During epidemics of obesity and type 2 diabetes, caloric increases have been due almost entirely to increased carbohydrates.

3. The benefits of dietary carbohydrate restriction do not require weight loss.

4. Although weight loss is not required for benefit, no dietary intervention is better than carbohydrate restriction for weight loss.

5. Adherence to low-carbohydrate diets in people with type 2 diabetes is at least as good as adherence to any other dietary interventions and is frequently significantly better.

6. Replacement of carbohydrate with protein is generally beneficial.

7. Dietary total and saturated fat do not correlate with risk of cardiovascular disease.

8. Saturated fatty acids in the blood are controlled by dietary carbohydrate more than by dietary lipids.

9. The best predictor of microvascular complications (kidney disease, nerve damage and damage to the retina in the eye) and, to a lesser extent, macrovascular complications (hardening of the arteries, angina, heart attack, skin ulcers, tissue death and stroke) in people with type 2 diabetes, is glycaemic control (determined in blood tests from levels of HbA1c, which measures how much sugar is attached to haemoglobin).

10. Dietary carbohydrate restriction is the most effective method (other than starvation) of reducing blood triglyceride levels and increasing HDL (good) cholesterol.

11. People with type 2 diabetes on carbohydrate-restricted diets reduce and frequently eliminate medication. People with type 1 usually require lower insulin doses.

12. Intensive glucose lowering through dietary carbohydrate restriction has no side effects comparable to those arising from intensive pharmacological treatment.

Dr Sarah Hallberg from Indiana University manages a medical weight-loss program, based on carbohydrate restriction. This program runs in complete contrast to the American Diabetes Association (ADA) diabetes management program. Noting that type 2 diabetes has traditionally been approached as 'a disease that will progress over time requiring increased oral medications and eventual insulin therapy', Dr Hallberg decided to place a group of 50 patients on the Indiana University low-carbohydrate medical weight-loss program and another group of 50 patients on the standard ADA program and see what happened.

The results were startling. The Indiana University medical diet was more effective than the ADA diet in weight loss and improvement in several markers of metabolic health. While HbA1c decreased in both groups, insulin usage dropped significantly among the Indiana University diet participants. Hallberg notes substantial cost savings would be available to patients on the Indiana University diet, as many of them decreased or eliminated medications for glycaemic control, hypertension (high blood pressure), cholesterol and gastric reflux.

Dr Richard Bernstein is a vibrant and healthy 81-year-old New York GP who developed type 1 diabetes at the age of twelve. Despite diligently following doctor's orders, Bernstein's suffered years of complications and fatigue, and his overall health began to deteriorate by his thirties. After his wife, also a doctor, obtained one of the new blood-glucose monitors for him, he began to monitor his blood glucose five times a day. Having noticed that his blood glucose fluctuated wildly after consumption of carbohydrates, he pursued a low-carbohydrate diet (the very opposite of what the ADA recommends) and was able to normalise his blood glucose and regain much of his health.

Dr Bernstein, wanting to share his information with the diabetic community, wrote a paper about his success with the diet, but the medical community refused to publish it as at that time he was an engineer, not a medical doctor. Bernstein responded by entering medical school in 1979 at the age of 45, then opening his own diabetes-oriented medical practice in 1983. Bernstein has achieved tremendous success with his low-carbohydrate diet, which bans or restricts all foods with added sugar or honey, all foods made from grains and grain flours, starchy vegetables such as potato, fruits and their juices, and all dairy except butter, cream and certain cheeses.

In 2010, at the age of 75 and having been a type 1 diabetic for more than 60 years, Bernstein continues in excellent health, with good kidney function and cholesterol levels. When he was 74, Bernstein also decided to have a calcium score test. The test involves taking a high-speed photograph of the heart so that the number of calcium deposits, as an indicator of hardening of the arteries, can be determined. Calcium scores can range from zero to 1000, good to bad. Dr Bernstein scored one. He credits the low-carbohydrate diet, which maintains normal blood glucose, and exercise including weight lifting and cycling on an exercise bike as the keys to his success.

After decades of working with diabetic patients, Bernstein strongly opposes the low-fat, high-carbohydrate diets recommended by the ADA. He has written numerous books on the subject, including his bestseller *Dr Bernstein's Diabetes Solution*, and continues to present his free online Diabetes University and videos.

Dr Jason Fung, a Canadian kidney specialist who was tired of sending his patients for limb amputations and dialysis treatment and never seeing them get any better, launched the Intensive Dietary Management Program with the aim of treating not diabetes but insulin resistance. Fung insists that because insulin resistance is a dietary disease, it demands a dietary response. Using a program that involves the ancient practice of intermittent fasting and modern-day carbohydrate restriction, Fung's team has helped many people lose weight and reverse their type 2 diabetes. His patients are charged a nominal fee of CA$100 for six months' participation in the program, demonstrating how inexpensive diabetes reversal can be. Many of his patients have been able to dramatically reduce or completely eliminate their medications, enabling further cost savings to them and to Canadian taxpayers. His blog, online lectures and book recommendations are useful for people who cannot attend his clinic but may want to pursue a diabetes-reversal program with their own doctor. Dr Fung's book *The Obesity Code* was published in 2016.

Alongside the new wave of doctors providing radical dietary solutions to their patients' diet-related health problems, is a large and growing movement of people across the West who are embarking on the low-carb lifestyle in order to get their metabolic syndrome or type 2 diabetes into remission. The low-carb movement has reached such epic proportions that followers can now go on low-carb ocean cruises, attend low-carb meetings and conferences around the world, listen to dedicated low-carb podcasts, read low-carb blogs and join online low-carb communities.

LOW-CARB IS NOTHING NEW: THE BANTING DIET

William Banting, born in 1797, was an upper middle-class funeral director from London whose family was famous for holding the royal warrant for state burials for five generations. Banting struggled with his weight and health for many years, and had tried numerous diets and popular remedies to no avail. His portly frame and boil-covered skin rendered him subject to the sneers and sniggers of strangers on the street; his shame and embarrassment led him to avoid socialising and using public transport. In desperation, he even tried a starvation diet, and yet he continued to gain weight. Rigorous exercise such as brisk walking and rowing only gave Banting a larger appetite.

In what was to become a turning point for Banting, he stumbled upon a Dr Harvey, who had an interest in 'corpulence', having just attended a lecture in Paris by Monsieur Claude Bernard on the subject of diet and diabetes. Harvey was keen to experiment with Bernard's ideas and a desperate Banting, having exhausted all other options, was more than willing to go along with it. Dr Harvey banned bread, milk, butter, sugar, beer and potatoes in the belief that food containing sugar and starch created fatness.

The new diet prescribed by Dr Harvey, but developed by Monsieur Bernard included beef, mutton, kidneys, broiled fish, bacon or cold meat, black tea or coffee and a 30-gram piece of toast for breakfast; fish, meat, vegetables (above ground only), 30-gram piece of toast, poultry or game, fruit, claret or sherry for lunch; cooked fruit, a rusk and black tea for afternoon tea; and meat or fish similar to lunch for dinner, along with a nightcap if required of gin, whisky, brandy or claret.

Banting was at first concerned that he would not have enough to eat on the new diet, but upon commencing the plan found that he had more than enough. He was also surprised that he was in fact benefiting in both mind and body. So impressed was he with his weight loss and incredible return to health and vitality that he self-published a pamphlet, the famous *Letter on Corpulence* in 1864, which he distributed at cost to himself but free to others. Banting could scarcely have imagined that his self-published pamphlet would one day be available to the world via the internet.

Banting desperately wanted the medical world to avail itself of this knowledge so that it could help people lose weight, recover their health and stop the torment of 'corpulence', but being a funeral director rather than a scientist he was unable to back up his claims with the hard scientific evidence and, like Dr Richard Bernstein, wasn't taken seriously.

Nevertheless, the Banting diet has been practised around the world for well over 200 years with similar success – some even know it as the Atkins Diet. So popular was the low-carbohydrate diet that people would say they were 'banting' rather than dieting.

The argument from vested interests

If the low-carb diet works so well for type 2 diabetes, why has it never become part of the official treatment for the reversal of the disease and its concomitant health consequences? After all, the low-fat, high-carbohydrate diet and exercise advice that has been the default position for type 2 diabetes 'treatment' during the global explosion of the disease has long been known to increase the risk of obesity, type 2 diabetes and cardiovascular problems. Until recently, the reason for the stony silence has been known only to the diet aristocracy. But in October 2015, Pamela Dyson, dietitian and CEO of the United Kingdom's Oxford Health Alliance, an organisation created with the objective of 'preventing and reducing the global impact of epidemic chronic disease', published a review that shed some interesting light on the matter.

According to Dyson, 'concern' has been raised that low-carbohydrate diets might be harmful to people with type 2 diabetes. She doesn't cite any proven mechanisms of how a low-carb approach can be harmful, but it is difficult to imagine that lowering carbohydrates could be much worse than the obesity, amputations, blindness, dialysis, cancer, physical and mental suffering, family break-up, poverty and early death already suffered by many of these patients.

A second major concern of both Dyson and her dietitian colleagues is the issue of what the UN's Food and Agriculture Organization calls 'sustainable nutrition'. Dyson notes that cereals such as wheat, sugar and seed oils are the least carbon-intensive crops to produce. But is this reason enough to allow these products to dominate the food supply, irrespective of any negative externalities? She also notes that low-carbohydrate diets promote foods such as vegetables, fruit, dairy and meat, whose production is evidently more carbon-intensive and may result in more greenhouse gas emissions. The implication seems to be that healthy, nutrient-dense eating could destroy the planet. In contrast, however, environmentalists say food wastage is a genuine threat to the climate. An estimated 30–40 per cent of food winds up in land-fill, where it emits the greenhouse gas methane and contributes to climate change.

Dyson suggests there is a risk that low-carb diets for diabetes could be seen as elitist, but surely we can't imagine that ampu-tations, blindness and dialysis are the best way to keep the rank and file grounded, and in my view we are all entitled to have good health irrespective of our social standing. She also notes that by 2030, 10 per cent of the world's population will have type 2 diabetes, which could be seen as an admission of failure on the part of the dietetics profession.

While Dyson declared no conflict of interest in the paper (a statement revised within the month), a quick check on The Oxford Health Alliance website reveals the charity organisation was formed as an actual alliance between the University of Oxford and the pharmaceutical company Novo Nordisk (UK and Australia), which specialises in diabetes medications. Other funding partners include:

- PepsiCo and PepsiCo Foundation
- Nestlé
- Johnson & Johnson
- Kissman Langford (a public relations firm specialising in damage control)
- Sudler & Hennessey (a healthcare marketing and communications company whose website boasts 'Proudly pushing drugs for 75 years')
- Diabetes Australia (whose corporate partners include Abbott Diabetes Care, AstraZeneca Diabetes, Bayer, Lilly Diabetes, Pharmaco Diabetes, Roche and Sanofi Diabetes)
- Cancer Council Australia
- Stroke Foundation, Australia (whose corporate partners include Bayer Australia, Bristol-Myers Squibb and Pfizer Alliance, Boehringer Ingelheim and Allergan)
- Heart Foundation, Australia (industry-funded and co-funded in partnership with Diabetes Australia)

- New South Wales Health Department
- University of Sydney.

Dyson concludes her review by announcing, contradictorily, that while low-carb diets seem to be safe and effective for those with diabetes, she suggests that other non-specific but sustainable diets are also available. In a later paper published by Dyson addressing arguments put forward by diet 'activists' regarding saturated fat and type 2 diabetes, Dyson noted that she has personally received honoraria for lectures from Abbott Diabetes Care, Lilly, MSD (Merck), Novo Nordisk, Janssen and Sanofi, in addition to unrestricted grants from Abbot Laboratories, the Sugar Bureau, the PepsiCo Foundation and Novo Nordisk. This is not to suggest that such industry connections would in any way influence Dyson's views, but rather speaks to the general ties that seem to exist between the dietetics and nutrition fields and big business – an issue the public is becoming increasingly aware of and that is explored further in the next chapter.

Sugar and wheat: more lethal in combination

In this and the previous two chapters we have seen, and just as Weston Price's indigenous groups found, that regular consumption of sugar and not just refined wheat but whole wheat can play a major role in the onset of serious health problems. The question now is which is guiltier: fructose, wheat or both?

Perhaps the answer can be found in a very small and seemingly insignificant study published in 2013. Two researchers, looking for new insights into metabolic syndrome and on the hunt for mainstream medical, complementary and alternative therapies for controlling or curing symptoms of the condition, decided to develop a new rat model that would most closely resemble metabolic syndrome, for use in studies of the condition. To this end, they fed four groups of rats different diets:

1. a regular diet with whole-wheat flour
2. a regular diet with refined wheat flour
3. a 60 per cent fructose diet with whole-wheat flour
4. a 60 per cent fructose diet with refined wheat flour.

The last group developed symptoms of metabolic syndrome in just four weeks, the fastest of any of the groups. The researchers also noted that replacing whole-wheat flour with refined flour induces more metabolic abnormalities, including low HDL cholesterol. In addition, this diet resulted in high blood pressure, high blood insulin, high blood glucose and a reduction in HDL cholesterol levels at four weeks, with endothelial dysfunction (an early stage in hardening of the arteries and coronary artery disease) at eight weeks.

It would seem that the more sugar and refined carbohydrate (or any carbohydrate for those who appear to have lost tolerance) we consume, the more sickness we can expect, and the more medications and hospital admissions we will require. The most recent Australian Health Survey (2011–12) revealed that Australians were consuming an average of 229 grams of carbohydrate per day (an amount considered high by Richard Feinman and his colleagues), drawing around 45 per cent of their total daily energy from carbohydrate, 24 per cent of which came from starch (mostly from wheat products) and 20 per cent from sugars. The Dietitians Association of Australia (DAA) suggests that 45 per cent should be the lower end of our total daily intake from carbohydrate foods, but that anything up to 65 per cent could be considered healthy.

It's curious, then, that independent researchers from a range of scientific disciplines noted in 2015 that 'carbohydrate restriction is the single most effective intervention for *reducing all of the features of metabolic syndrome*' (my italics), better than all the blockbuster medications used to control symptoms of the condition. In 2013, the sales of diabetes drugs hit US$23 billion. (In an interesting aside, an article published in *The Guardian* in January 2016 discussed why pharmaceutical companies had reduced investment in the development of new drugs for psychiatric and neurological conditions by 70 per cent in the last decade. One of the experts the journalists interviewed suggested that the industry players decided it was easier to make money from cancer and diabetes.)

Sugar shenanigans

Many in-depth books have been written about the negative health implications of consuming sugar, refined grain and 'bad' fat; the last three chapters have simply provided an overview – and an invitation to learn more by following up the references I have cited. The medical and scientific researchers I have named specifically are among a small number of people who live and breathe these subjects, and yet their knowledge has until recently been kept from the general public by various filtering organisations that tightly control the narrative to the detriment of that public. This unfortunate situation is thankfully changing as the public becomes more questioning and cynical about what we have been told about diet and health over the last 50 years. And living in the information age, we are no longer reliant on a single source of health and diet information or on trips to a university library, and scientific researchers and doctors can now come forward and share their knowledge and experience with us directly.

The last word in this series of chapters goes to John Yudkin, the man who first tried to draw our attention to the possible health problems associated with sugar and carbohydrates, and had his personal and professional reputation destroyed for his efforts. In the most recent edition of Yudkin's book, a new final chapter from the author gives a very detailed account of the lengths the food industry went to ensure the public was never informed about his team's research or in fact any research regarding the risks associated with sugar consumption.

Perhaps his most revealing insight into industry tactics is his detailed account of the birth in 1967 of the British Nutrition Foundation (BNF), an organisation initially funded by the sugar refiners Tate & Lyle and the wheat-flour refiners Rank. Both Tate & Lyle and Rank shared common business goals and interests, and there were also personal friendships between the two families. Yudkin reveals that the BNF initially struggled to obtain financial support for its various activities from the wider processed-food industry, until, in a stroke of genius, its director, Professor Alastair Frazer, alerted industry players to increased consumer concern about processes and additives used by the rapidly expanding processed-food industry.

To counter the issue, Professor Frazer suggested that the BNF would act as a 'protective fence' between the industry and the general public. In other words, the BNF became a 'gatekeeper' that would stand between not just the public and the food industry, but the public and the scientific community as well. From that point on, the British public would know only what the BNF decided it should know. In the ensuing years, a 'community' of filtering not-for-profit organisations would appear in Western nations, spanning not just nutrition and dietetics, but organs and diseases as well. The most incredible aspect of the rise of the filtering community is that not one disease or condition has been eradicated as a result of their efforts. In fact, the opposite has occurred – diseases have exploded across the board and been exported around the world. Perhaps it's time we looked further into the collective raison d'être of these organisations.

Today, corporate membership of the BNF reads like a who's who of the processed-food industry, and it's difficult to imagine it would be able to play a leading role in the fight against food-related diseases when doing so might negatively impact the financial position or reputation of its own sponsors.

Yudkin's final chapter is also one of the most comprehensively detailed accounts of the unrelenting attacks upon the work, personal integrity and professional reputation of a scientist at the hands of industry interests (in this case, from the sugar industry), ever written. The savaging of individual scientists who dare to challenge the official narrative is nothing new, and we see the same thing happening to scientists who challenge the safety of other products linked to the chemicals industry, such as cigarettes, pharmaceuticals, organophosphates and foods containing GMOs.

This phenomenon, known as pseudoscepticism, essentially involves 'manufacturing doubt' by way of perpetually muddying the research waters in order to cause confusion and controversy among the scientific community, policymakers and the general public alike. The playbook of pseudoscepticism has been recycled by several industries, which resort to the same low tactics every time. These follow a very predictable pattern, involving unrelenting denials or trivialising the problem followed by calls for more evidence. When evidence is produced, the data is cherry-picked by industry interests, the blame is shifted, the scientists and their work attacked. In addition, industry-friendly scientists are hired and front groups created. The art and practice of pseudoscepticism is detailed in the 2010 book *Merchants of Doubt* by historians Naomi Oreskes and Erik Conway. Pseudoscepticism is a big problem for the legitimate scientists who are trying to protect citizens from the worst excesses of industry, and nowhere is it more prevalent than in today's food industry.

Yudkin's unyielding belief that the 'freedom of choice exists only if there is freedom of information' motivated him to continue his work under the enormous pressure brought to bear by those who stood to lose the most. Like the abolitionists before him, Yudkin came to understand two things: that suffering and human lives count for little when it comes to profit; and that the interests controlling the processed-food industry don't give up easily.

8

The diet wars

In 2011, the then US Secretary of State Hillary Clinton appeared before the Foreign Policy Priorities Committee to defend the budget of the State Department. She was famously captured on the public-service cable channel C-SPAN delivering her blunt assessment: 'We are in an *information war* and we are losing that war.' She was of course referring to the rise of Al-Jazeera and Russia Today as credible threats to US propaganda efforts both at home and abroad. By 2016, Clinton was not just battling an information war in her election battle with Donald Trump, but an *information race*. Only this time she was dealing with the drudgereport.com, the number two ranked media publisher in the United States after MSN and reputedly run by just four people. The real issue that plagued Clinton, however, was how to deal with an increasingly fragmented non-corporate-controlled media. What happens when you can no longer monopolise information? What happens when newspeak doesn't cut it anymore? And worse – what happens when nobody's listening?

But Clinton hasn't been alone in grappling with a loss of relevancy among those she seeks to influence. Institutions across the board are suddenly finding themselves continually under siege, and health-sector filtering organisations such as the DAA and the Australian Heart Foundation, which have traditionally controlled the 'what we eat' space, are no exception. The battle for relevancy is being fought on both social media and in bookshops around the country, as everyone from mummy bloggers to media identities, models, doctors, lawyers, chefs, scientists, actors, surgeons and singers bring new ideas and alternative points of view about what we eat and how we eat it. Michael Pollan, in his book *In Defence of Food*, momentarily cut through the noise and sensibly told us to 'Eat food. Not too much. Mostly plants' before being drowned out by the clatter of disruption. So who are these diet insurgents, and why have they risen in such numbers and with such forcible opposition to mainstream dietary and health orthodoxy?

The rise of the micropowers

In his 2013 book *The End of Power*, Moisés Naím discusses the rise of the 'micropowers' that seem to emerge from nowhere to shake up the old order, their strength derived precisely from exploiting their rivals' weaknesses. Micropowers are authentic, nimble, tech and social-media savvy, and unconstrained by politics, the need to follow an established party line or expectations of industry backers.

These 'digital Davids . . . wear down, impede, undermine, sabotage and outflank' the clumsy, disorganised and confused 'Goliaths'. Micropowers are able to pull back the curtain and, like Toto in *The Wizard of Oz*, expose the noticeable flaws and dubious conflicts of interest underpinning the established order, publicly skewering the Goliaths at every turn. With potentially millions of social-media followers, the reach of the micropowers' message cannot be underestimated or easily thwarted, not even by an army of paid 'scientific experts' possessed of a clear strategic intent to muddy the waters. It's bad news all round for the Goliaths – the micropowers are just getting started.

The traditional 'diet experts' and their corporate connections have been hit hard by diet and wellness micropowers, and on the surface it's not hard to see why. While the old order desperately clings to the same confusing and counterintuitive messages that helped create the chronic-disease mess, the micropowers are confronting the problem head on, simultaneously educating an increasingly desperate public while supporting their stance with the help of open-access scientific literature and fiercely independent medical and nutrition experts.

The diet insurgents have spotted the gap in the market – the difference between what the scientific community knows contributes to chronic disease and what filtering organisations funded by the processed-food industry, such as the DAA, bother telling us. The micropowers at this point appear to have the greatest chance of turning around the chronic-disease epidemic through a simple formula of education, engaged communities and solutions that are obviously working for people. The micropowers are not just filling the vacuum created by distracted 'diet experts' who bicker among themselves, dance around the issues and busily play food politics;

they are forcing a change in the narrative and openly challenging the status quo. At a minimum, the micropowers have been able to get consumers to rethink their diet and lifestyle choices in ways academia and health authorities could only dream of and, at their best, they are changing lives for the better.

Recent Australian battles

An example of just how pervasive health micropowers have become and how rattled the old order appears in trying to negate the micropowers' spreading influence, is the tug-of-war that began in Australia in 2008 when 'recovering corporate lawyer' David Gillespie published his seminal book *Sweet Poison*, which became a bestseller. Gillespie's total sales for health-focused books have surpassed the 230,000 copies mark. Gillespie attracted significant media coverage of his journey from obese father trying numerous diets to lose weight to his decision to cut out sugar, losing 40 kilograms in the process. Gillespie's weight loss and reclaimed health were extraordinary and worthy of praise in any doctor's book, yet by far the harshest criticism of both Gillespie and his message came from the 'diet expert' community itself, and the loudest voices emanated from Sydney University.

In 2013, nutritionist Bill Shrapnel, then of the University of Sydney's Nutrition Research Foundation, was quoted in the *Sydney Morning Herald* claiming that the data linking sugar to health problems was 'poor' and dismissed the war on sugar. Shrapnel was one of fourteen health experts named by Coca-Cola in March 2016 as having been a financial beneficiary of its funding in 2013 for his role as facilitator at a symposium. Shrapnel runs a nutrition blog, and, according to his own biography, consults to industry lobby groups such as Sugar Australia, the Australian Beverages Council and the Australian Food and Grocery Council, and processed-food companies such as Kellogg Australia and Goodman Fielder.

In 2011, Sarah Wilson, who was already a media personality, documented her account of going sugar-free on her blog, having been inspired by reading David Gillespie's book. Wilson's story of failing health and path to recovery hit a nerve with consumers and she became a media sensation. In 2012, her book *I Quit Sugar* sold more than 100,000 copies and spawned an empire that now employs thirteen people and turns over AU$1.8 million annually. Wilson's eight-week program claims to have helped more than 600,000 people turn their weight and health around.

In 2012, Wilson was featured on the television program *60 Minutes* alongside anti-sugar endocrinologist and professor of paediatrics Professor Robert Lustig, discussing the health risks associated with sugar. Providing the counterpoint to Lustig and Wilson was University of Sydney nutrition professor Jennie Brand-Miller, co-author of the widely cited and controversial 2011 paper 'The Australian paradox' published in *Nutrition* under Brand-Miller's guest editorship. The peer-reviewed paper, co-authored by Dr Alan Barclay, the Australian Diabetes Council's head of research, claimed that unlike other countries around the world, Australians were eating less sugar while obesity had increased, and concluded, 'The findings challenge the implicit assumption that taxes and other measures to reduce intake of soft drinks will be an effective strategy in global efforts to reduce obesity.'

Based upon these conclusions, the paper was unsurprisingly seized upon by the Australian Beverages Council in a formal submission to the National Health Medical Research Council Dietary Guidelines Committee to counter a call in the draft dietary guidelines for a reduction in the consumption of sugary foods and drinks. The study was also used by the Australian Beverages Council in a submission to the Victoria's Citizens' Jury on Obesity to denounce soft-drink taxes as 'ineffective, inefficient and unfair for a range of reasons'. The Australian Beverages Council along with the Australian Grocery Council, is on the Steering Group of the Citizens' Jury.

One person who took exception to the factual accuracy and public-health implications of the paper was banking economist and statistics buff Rory Robertson. Having spent years knee-deep in data, Robertson raised several concerns with Sydney University. An independent review was held and Robertson's complaint was broken down into three key issues:

1. the content of the paper – discrepancies in the statistical data
2. the authorship of the paper – omission as an author of a masters student who is acknowledged as having done the research
3. conflicts of interest – pertaining to Brand-Miller's connections to the sugar industry via her role as director of the Glycemic Index Foundation, a 'not-for-profit University of Sydney spin-off company', and Barclay's connections to the Australian Diabetes Council, the Glycemic Index Foundation and Coca-Cola. (The Glycemic Index Foundation charges food manufacturers a fee to feature its 'Low GI' logo on certain foods such as CSR's LoGICane

sugar, canned fruit and jams, Kellogg's breakfast cereals and assorted mueslis, ice cream, breads and hot chocolate drinks. Alan Barclay was also named in 2016 as a recipient of Coca-Cola funding for his 2011 webinar.)

The investigation did not uphold all of Robertson's complaints (including those regarding conflicts of interest) but did raise the issue of publishing a 'big' public-policy result through a soft channel and recommended the authors publish a correction to errors in their data. More importantly, the investigation and media interest, including an investigation by ABC's Lateline screened in 2016, enabled significant insight into the normally hidden links between public-health academics charged with protecting the nation's health and the sugar and processed-food industry, as well as the issue of either real or perceived conflicts of interest. In this respect, members of the public have been able to read the documents and reach their own conclusions regarding the behaviour of these traditional health authorities. In an era where trust has become the name of the game, such revelations do little to help the diet expert's cause.

Bloodied but not bowed, the authors of 'The Australian paradox' still maintain that their figures demonstrate Australia's obesity crisis is about 'anything but the sugar'. In an interview with the *Sydney Morning Herald*, Brand-Miller insisted her stance was not related to commercial interests, but rather a measured 'expert opinion' based upon 35 years of experience and a 'sincere belief' that moderate amounts of sugar contribute to a healthy diet.

While this short history of the sugar tussle is not to suggest that any of the nutrition professionals mentioned are conflicted due to their industry links, the episode speaks to the growing public unease when ties between industry and public health academia come to light.

Gluten-free and Paleo

In 2013, health experts openly scratched their heads wondering why everyone was going gluten-free despite not having been medically advised to do so. Ultimately, gluten-free was officially declared a fad diet, a fashion statement confined to Sydney's exclusive suburbs. Prominent dietitian Rosemary Stanton announced that people who went gluten-free without testing did so to make themselves feel 'special', while the Grains and Legumes Nutrition Council (GLNC) nutritionist Michelle Broom alerted the gluten-free brigade to the much higher levels of salt and saturated fat in gluten-free food. (It's worth noting here that the GLNC, which refers to itself as the 'independent authority on the nutrition and health benefits of grains', at the time of writing listed among its financial 'contributors' Kellogg's, George Weston Foods, Goodman Fielder, Sanitarium, Bakers Delight and the Australian Food and Grocery Council.)

It turns out nobody bothered listening to Stanton or Broom. In April 2015, the GLNC reported that the gluten-free 'fad' (which *had* previously been confined to Sydney's exclusive suburbs) had unfortunately spread to the mainstream, resulting in a 30 per cent fall in grain consumption in just three years. Another code red was issued to not just the gluten-free brigade but also the Paleos that they could be missing out on vital fibre and nutrients (despite the core of the Paleo diet being high-fibre, nutrient-dense foods).

In 2014, a newly slimmed-down, happy and healthy-looking Pete Evans appeared on the popular television show *My Kitchen Rules* and put the grain, dairy, sugar and junk-food-free Paleo diet on the map for Australians. People were interested and gave it a go. Many felt that having 'tried everything' to lose weight or feel better, they had nothing to lose. Evans conducted national tours, drawing thousands of people from across the country, and his Paleo books sold more than 415,000 copies. His Facebook likes exploded from 100,000 to more than 1 million in one year, as followers posted victory report after victory report detailing their weight loss, dramatically improved blood test results and radically improved health. Paleo subsumed the 'gluten-free' narrative, spawning books, television shows, cafés and food products.

In July 2014, the DAA issued a media release calling the pesticide/herbicide-free vegetable, fruit, grass-fed meat, nut, seed and water Paleo diet 'potentially dangerous'. The evidence cited for the 'danger' appeared to be fewer than ten studies, conducted over three months or less and involving very few participants. It's curious to me that an organisation that claims to provide evidence-based information could denounce an eating style as dangerous based upon virtually no evidence.

The DAA receives financial support from processed-food companies such as Arnott's, Australia's top manufacturer of sugar- and wheat-containing biscuits. Another sponsor, US-owned Campbell Soup Company (which also owns Arnott's), has been criticised for the levels of salt in its soups – the firm even stated at an investor meeting that it would boost the salt content of its US products to combat sluggish sales. Other sponsors and partnerships of the DAA have included Unilever, Nestlé and the Australian Grains and Legumes Nutrition Council.

The 'dangerous' claims were followed by a humorous declaration from a News Limited writer that Paleo was 'un-Australian', an ironic statement given the diet of our Indigenous population (among others) was, for tens of thousands of years, hunter-gatherer – in other words Paleo. It was only when they were given grains, sugar and seed oil that their health, communities and future were destroyed. And as we have seen, when nutrition researcher Kerin O'Dea returned some Indigenous Australians to their traditional hunter-gatherer diet, several were able to recover their health.

The nutrition 'experts'

The DAA issued numerous media releases, 'hot topic' releases and media rebuttals during 2014 and 2015 designed to dampen the effects of the micropowers. In 2015, it issued a 'hot topic' release effectively rebutting the documentary *That Sugar Film*, Australia's highest grossing local documentary film on record. Australian actor and director Damon Gameau, a 'clean-food' eater who had not partaken of processed foods or added sugar for three years, consumed over a two-month period the equivalent of 40 teaspoons of added sugar per day, from processed foods marketed as 'healthy' or 'low-fat', such as yoghurt and breakfast cereals. By the end of his experiment, Gameau had gained 10 centimetres of fat around his waist, reported feeling sick and experienced mood swings. Respected chemical pathologist and chair of the International Federation of Clinical Chemistry Committee on Analytical Quality, Dr Ken Sikaris, told Gameau he had signs of fatty liver disease, noting that it was the first time he had seen the condition develop in two to three weeks. Dr Sikaris's observation regarding non-alcoholic fatty liver disease was most intriguing, as media reports have noted a homegrown epidemic of this condition – one in three Australians, some as young as twenty, now show symptoms. The endpoint for this disease is a liver transplant or death.

While health campaigners such as Jamie Oliver applauded the film, the DAA said it was 'simplistic and unhelpful' to blame sugar alone (which Gameau had not done) for Australia's obesity and health crisis. In addition, the DAA expressed disappointment that Gameau's documentary featured him consuming healthier foods such as sugary 'health' yoghurts and sugary 'health' breakfast cereals, because they contained not just added sugar but valuable nutrients.

Contrast the actions of the DAA with that of the Heart and Stroke Foundation of Canada, which in June 2014 issued a media release announcing the end of its Health Check program, including the ubiquitous 'Tick' on processed foods in addition to the processed-food-industry money that came with it. Having terminated the program because 'much has changed in the past 15 years in the world of food and nutrition', the foundation subsequently published a damning position statement titled 'Sugar, heart disease and stroke', citing the body of available evidence that excess sugar consumption is linked to poor health, including heart disease, stroke, diabetes, high blood cholesterol, cancer and dental caries and recommending the introduction of a sugar tax. The statement asserted that the Canadian government should avoid public-health partnerships with producers and suppliers of foods high in free sugars. (As we will see later in this chapter, the Australian Heart Foundation terminated its Tick program in December 2015.)

Dietitians in general fly under the public's radar. In a 2008 national survey conducted in the United States by the prestigious

Institute for the Future in Palo Alto, on behalf of Coca-Cola, dietitians and nutritionists were ranked last by consumers (35 per cent) as an information source for buying food or health products. Indeed, consumers obtained their nutritional information via a product label (68 per cent), friend (52 per cent), doctor (41 per cent) or even health website (37 per cent) rather than a dietitian. This should come as no surprise in light of a discovery made by the online group Ninjas for Health. In 2015, Coca-Cola published a list of diet experts, doctors and scientists with whom its employees routinely 'collaborate and consult' and who had been funded to the tune of US$2.3 million in the past five years. An analysis by the Ninjas for Health noted that by far the largest group of collaborators is dietitians (57 per cent) followed by academics (20 per cent) and medical professionals (7 per cent), with a few fitness experts, chefs and authors thrown in. These experts were given money for travel and related expenses, and professional fees. Many of the dietitians appeared to be members of the US Academy of Nutrition and Dietetics. Perhaps reflecting increasingly deep divisions within the field of dietetics and nutrition, a group called Dietitians for Professional Integrity has formed in the United States. The dietitians involved are fed up with what they perceive as too much influence over their profession from food companies.

In 2015, Coca-Cola UK announced a similar list of collaborators from the British nutrition and medical world. While three funding recipients refused to have their names made public, they, in addition to a further 27 individuals received a total of £355,453 for travel, related expenses and professional fees during the period 2010–15. Of the 27 named, thirteen were prominent dietitians while the remainder were a mix of doctors, psychologists, scientists, a pharmacologist and a dentist. All were prominent in the field of public health.

The consumers' viewpoint

As the official 'what to eat' institutions struggle to understand, come to terms with or even respond logically to their diminishing ability to influence an increasingly sceptical and angry public, perhaps it's time to genuinely consider why consumers might identify more with a micropower, doctor or even the neighbour's cat over a 'registered practising dietitian'.

1. Fear and experience

As demonstrated earlier, Weston Price's indigenous groups were fully aware that the foods introduced to their diets did, on some level, negatively impact their immunity, rendering them susceptible to disease, infertility, deformities and early death. Many were also aware that a return to a nutrient-dense, traditional diet, irrespective of the components of that diet, could offer them an escape from physical breakdown and a return to good health.

It could be argued that we are in a similar situation today. In 2017, it would seem that we all know somebody who has either battled with or lost their life to cancer in one or other of its many forms. We either suffer ourselves or know somebody who suffers from an autoimmune disease such as thyroiditis, coeliac disease, allergies, rheumatoid arthritis, multiple sclerosis, psoriasis, eczema or one of the numerous other autoimmune conditions. Many of us also know somebody whose child has autism, somebody with metabolic syndrome or type 2 diabetes, and somebody with depression. We seem to be surrounded by sickness. It's not going away and we are worried. That this situation has unfolded under the watch of a cadre of health and diet organisations has not gone unnoticed and is deeply worrying to many of us.

While the most publicly derided and controversial aspect of the diet–disease spectrum involves bloggers – such as Belle Gibson – proffering unsubstantiated claims of curing (either real or imagined) cancer through diet and wellness protocols while turning a tidy profit in the process, there are also many genuine quiet achievers.

In this 'space in the middle' we find the soccer mum who lost 5 kilograms and largely weaned her children from all the sugar they were eating by reading Sarah Wilson's books or taking them to see *That Sugar Film*. We find the overweight grandmother staring down the barrel of type 2 diabetes, possible limb amputation and kidney failure, who, with the help of an understanding doctor and a copy of *Wheat Belly*, elected to stare down her metabolic syndrome instead (sparing an overburdened medical system and the taxpayer in the process). We find the young lady suffering from MS who was able to rid herself of migraines, depression and severe MS symptoms by reading about Dr Terry Wahl's journey of overcoming the disease and embarking on similar life changes. We find the obese and depressed mother who has tried and tried to lose weight on a high-carbohydrate, low-fat diet then finally achieves weight-loss success by 'going Paleo' with Pete Evans, and is overjoyed at being a healthy and energetic parent for the first time.

In this space, we find scores of people sharing their journeys from various debilitating conditions to either much-improved or full health. To suggest they are *all* fabricating their stories is laughable. To suggest they should continue to suffer in silence and 'wait for the science to ripen' before changing their habits is odious, given the blatant lack of political will or research funding available for such endeavours. To advise them to snap out of it and immediately return to the latest incarnation of the carbohydrate-loaded food pyramid demonstrates a woeful understanding of the desperate situation with which so many are grappling. The one-size-fits-all high-carbohydrate, low-fat diet sold to us by health institutions as promoting 'all-round' health simply does not match our experience as the toll from food-based disease continues to mount. The idea that we are not allowed to question these failed policies in the light of what is happening seems truly an insult to an intelligent, educated and informed populace.

2. The rise of allergies, food intolerances and autoimmune diseases

According to a 2013 report from the Australasian Society of Clinical Immunology and Allergy (ASCIA), allergies and immune diseases are among the fastest growing chronic diseases in Australia. In addition, around 10 per cent of Australian infants have a proven food allergy, one of the highest incidences in the world. In 2005 the cost to the economy of allergic diseases alone was estimated to be AU$30 billion. The number of allergy sufferers is projected to increase by 70 per cent to 7.7 million by 2050.

Almost 20 per cent of Australians have an allergy that involves the immune system reacting to a particular food, resulting in dizziness, nausea, vomiting, rash, itchy skin, eyes, throat or tongue, swelling or potentially life-threatening anaphylaxis. The most common allergens are eggs, gluten (in wheat, rye and barley), milk, fish, peanuts, crustaceans, soybeans, tree nuts, sesame seeds and sulfites. Of particular concern is that food-induced anaphylaxis has doubled in the last ten years, with hospital admissions increasing fourfold in the last twenty years.

Food intolerance is understood to affect more people than food allergy, although exact numbers are difficult to gauge. Food intolerance is an inability to digest a particular food, and symptoms can involve bloating, gassiness, runny nose, stomach ache and diarrhoea. Foods mostly involved in intolerance include milk, gluten, food additives and sulfites.

According to the Australian Bureau of Statistics, in 2011–12, 17 per cent of Australians (approximately 3.7 million people) aged two years and over reported avoiding certain foods due to allergy or intolerance. The most commonly cited type of food intolerances were dairy (4.5 per cent) and gluten (2.5 per cent). Long-time restaurateur Gail Donovan raised the issue of allergies and intolerances in 2016, noting that food intolerances have been the biggest thing to hit the restaurant world in the last two years. Donovan revealed that at least half of all diners in the twenty to 30 age bracket will have allergies or intolerances to certain foods.

People suffering from any of these conditions must find ways to avoid consuming the offending foods. At the consumer end, this ultimately translates into expanding markets for both fresh and convenience 'free-from' foods and recipe books. The 'free-from' market has grown year on year, reflecting the rising number of people being diagnosed with or themselves becoming aware of food intolerances and allergies. According to market research firm Euromonitor, the global 'free-from' market was projected to grow from US$9.1 billion in 2011 to US$13.2 billion by 2015, with gluten- and lactose/dairy-free foods substantially outperforming the diabetic category.

On the home-cooking front, the Paleo diet in particular may be convenient to people in this category, as its default position is strict avoidance of key allergens such as grains, dairy, soybeans, processed foods and food additives. Paleo involves home cooking using unprocessed ingredients, and allows allergy/intolerance sufferers to enjoy greater confidence in avoiding trigger foods.

Autoimmunity could be considered a silent epidemic, as despite little funding and scant media coverage, it's a rapidly growing problem. More than 130 different diseases come under the auto-immunity umbrella, including coeliac disease (see page 177), dermatitis herpetiformis (see page 178), autoimmune thyroid diseases (Hashimoto's and Grave's), vitiligo, psoriasis, rheuma-toid and psoriatic arthritis, Crohn's disease, ulcerative colitis, type 1 diabetes, multiple and systemic sclerosis, Addison's disease, autoimmune neuropathy, alopecia areata, systemic lupus erythe-matosus, Sjögren's syndrome, polymyalgia rheumatica and chronic active hepatitis to name but a few (for a full list, see the appendix).

Individually, these conditions would appear to affect small numbers compared to heart disease, cancer and diabetes, but according to ASCIA, autoimmunity is more common than cancer or heart disease and, according to some in the field of autoim-munology, is the third leading cause of death globally. Autoimmune disease frequently runs in families but can manifest in different ways and at different ages. It disproportionately affects women and significantly affects quality of life and ability to earn an income, disrupts family and social life, and in many cases results in years lost to disability.

While the exact pathogenesis for food-related autoimmune diseases is unclear (except in the case of coeliac disease and dermatitis herpetiformis), researchers recognise the role of both genetic and environmental factors, including dietary antigens, infectious agents and environmental toxins (such as herbicides and pesticides), and their possible impact on the gut microbiota (see page 84).

In addition to the role of genes and environmental factors is the issue of intestinal permeability. The noted paediatric gastroenterologist Alessio Fasano has studied and written extensively on the subject of intestinal permeability in relation to coeliac disease, and his team was the first to discover the key molecule named zonulin and its role in altering the barrier function of the gut (see page 181). Once this barrier function is compromised, foreign proteins are able to travel through the 'leaks' and journey to other tissues and organs inside the body, where they can inflict damage. Zonulin release is triggered by gluten-containing grains.

Given the possible role of intestinal permeability in many autoimmune diseases, it becomes easier to understand why numerous sufferers anecdotally report diminishing or permanent relief from symptoms on a gluten-free or Paleo-style diet. Clearly, more studies are urgently needed to determine the role of environmental food triggers in autoimmunity, to relieve both people of their suffering and strain on the health system.

Given that so many of us are now experiencing allergies, intolerances and autoimmunity, is it now time to consign standardised dietary advice to the annals of history? Can health institutions really continue to apply a one-size-fits-all model to an entire population when it would seem that the population is anything but standard?

3. One diet does not fit all

Perhaps one of the most important facts revealed by Weston Price's research is that no one diet fits everybody – a fact supported by modern-day research into genetics, epigenetics and the microbiome. One 2015 study demonstrated that there are profound differences in the way people respond to the same foods, and foods that elicit a healthy response (in terms of blood-glucose levels) for some, may provoke a dangerous response in others. The study involved connecting 800 non-diabetic Israeli individuals between the ages of eighteen and 70 to a continuous glucose monitor for seven days, ultimately recording more than 1.5 million glucose measurements. While connected, the participants recorded food intake, exercise and sleep in real time via smartphone. Stool samples for micro-biota sampling were also taken from the group.

Because the researchers used controlled settings for standard-ised meals, they were able to demonstrate that, contrary to popular belief, the glycemic index (GI) is not a set value or intrinsic prop-erty of the food, but is dependent upon an individual's response. For example, one participant recorded a spike in blood glucose after eating a banana (considered a low-GI food), yet their blood glucose remained stable after eating a biscuit (considered a high-GI food). Conversely, another participant recorded a spike after eating the same biscuit, yet recorded a lowering of blood glucose after eating a banana. One participant's blood-glucose levels spiked after eating tomatoes, considered both a health food and given a very low GI. Moreover, the authors demonstrated that the composition of the gut microbiota is significantly associated with the blood-glucose response after eating. Based upon their findings, the authors stressed the need for personalised nutrition plans over universal dietary advice, and expressed concern that nutritionally 'compliant' people may have been led down the road to metabolic syndrome and type 2 diabetes by dietary instructions that were not suited to them on an individual level, and were in fact potentially dangerous.

WHAT IS THE GLYCEMIC INDEX?

The glycemic index (GI) aims to rank foods according to their effect on blood glucose. It does so by measuring the total rise in blood glucose (in a test subject) after that food is eaten and comparing it with the rise caused by pure glucose. It's called an index because it doesn't use the actual figures obtained but ranks foods on a scale of zero to 100, where glucose is set at 100.

Critics point out that in order to test the GI of foods, those foods are eaten in isolation, which is rare in the real world, and that interaction with other foods can alter their effect on blood glucose. It also says nothing about the health or otherwise of the other nutrients in that food.

This finding naturally leads us to the propensity of the diet experts to refer to any diet other than their universal dietary advice as a 'fad diet'. The vast majority of the diets commonly referred to as fads in fact fail to qualify as any such thing. Many of these diets have been around for years and, in the case of the Banting diet, more than 100 years. Such staying power in terms of popularity means that they have long surpassed fad status, which in marketing terms is only a few months (a good example being the 'onesie' craze). Applying the 'fad' label is a way for traditional health authorities to diminish the value of different offerings while attempting to reclaim their rapidly waning expert authority. It's part of an information war that is all but lost. It could be argued that there is a *trend* towards certain eating styles, such as clean, low-carb, ketogenic (super low-carb) or Paleo, but the all-important *shift* is in favour of fresh foods that deliver health and vitality.

The reason for the popularity of different diets is that they please some of the people for some of the time – or indeed all of the time depending on what an individual may be trying to achieve with their health. When someone commits to a journey towards health and wellness, they by default must follow an arc of discovery until their health goals align with what works to achieve them – for some this is Paleo, for others low-carb and for others it will be something different again. A one-size-fits-all approach to food intake has never worked and will never work.

4. The role of the microbiome

A common feature of the newer class of 'clean' or 'wellness' diets, such as raw-food or Paleo, is that they address the health of the microbiome, and understand and respect its important role in keeping us healthy. Scientific evidence continues to mount regarding the importance of healthy gastrointestinal flora, supporting a concept and practice that has been commonplace in many cultures for thousands of years.

The most inexpensive way to have a positive impact on the microbiome appears to be via the regular use of raw and cultured vegetables, bone broths, organic yoghurt and kefir from grass-fed cows, coconut milk kefir and raw apple cider vinegar. Despite the mounting evidence regarding the importance of a healthy microbiome, most health institutions have thus far failed to address the issue.

Herbicides and pesticides routinely sprayed on our foods may harm important bacteria that inhabit our microbiome, possibly leading to the inability of gut flora to function properly and subsequent health problems. Clean-eating advocates cite this as one reason for purchasing organic foods where possible, as they are free of such chemicals.

In late 2015, I contacted Alessio Fasano to ask whether he stood by his 2009 assertion in *Scientific American* that a trio of factors underpinned 'most if not all' autoimmune diseases: an environmental substance, a genetic component and an unusually permeable gut. He replied that he did – but had two more ingredients to add to the recipe: an inappropriate response of the innate immune system, and an imbalanced gut microbiota.

5. Vested interests

In her opening address at the 8th Global Conference on Health Promotion in Finland, World Health Organization Director-General Margaret Chan pulled few punches regarding conflicts of interest with respect to food and health, describing the vested interests as 'not so friendly'. In her speech, Chan specifically noted that efforts to prevent chronic diseases sat diametrically at odds with the business interests of powerful economic players. Big Tobacco are no longer the only boys in town. Today we have Big Soda, Big Food and Big Alcohol – all industries that fear regulation and use front groups, lobbies, lawsuits, industry-funded research and promises of self-regulation to muddy the waters and confuse the public. Chan also noted that these players use gifts, grants and donations to worthy causes to boost their image, promote personal responsibility and decry government actions as an assault on freedom of choice. Chan used her speech to remind us all that not a single country in the world had managed to rein in its obesity epidemic in all age groups, noting that this situation was not a failure on the part of individual willpower but of political will to take on big business.

Consumers, too, have become increasingly suspicious of institutions that ostensibly exist to protect society's health while receiving patronage from various corporate interests whose ultimate raison d'être is to make profit and pursue growth. Many of us are now openly questioning why we should be taking health or nutrition advice from organisations that receive funding from processed-food manufacturers. And so we should. The very whisper of 'captured agencies' determining important aspects of our health makes us very uncomfortable in an era where the issue of trust is becoming paramount. Dubious examples continue to come to light of the behaviour of these very strange bedfellows.

Australia's most public and illuminating food-related conflict of interest case is that of Alastair Furnival, the former chief of staff to then Assistant Health Minister Fiona Nash, and his role in the removal from public view of a government healthy food ratings website (designed to assist consumers in making 'healthier' processed-food choices using the National Health Star Ratings scheme). Furnival had been co-principal of and still held shares in Australian Public Affairs, a lobbying business whose clients included food-processing firms affected by the healthy food ratings scheme. Given that the primary goal of lobbying entities is to minimise government-imposed business regulations, the appointment of Furnival to the very department charged with protecting the health of Australian taxpayers is nothing short of scandalous.

In addition, Australian Public Affairs had been placed under the control of a parent company, Strategic Issues Management, which was jointly owned by Furnival and his wife, Tracy Cain. This discovery led to his resignation. Further stories came to light about his role in stripping government funding from Australia's peak drug and alcohol body, the Alcohol and Other Drugs Council of Australia, which had worked for 46 years to minimise alcohol and drug harm to the Australian public. According to media reports, Australian Public Affairs seemed to have been involved in alcohol-industry PR as late as 2012, while the council's chief executive, David Templeman, noted that the industry had been unhappy with the council's advocacy, expressing as much to the chair of its board. Templeman also noted the powerful interests involved.

'Health advisor' Furnival was also found to have lobbied the Tasmanian government directly in 2012, before his appointment to the department, to secure taxpayer funds for chocolate manu-facturer Cadbury. In a move that could be attributed to either bad taste or breathtaking ignorance, Furnival was later photographed alongside Prime Minister Tony Abbott at the Pollie Pedal event in 2013, wearing (as were all the others) a jersey sponsored by AMGEN, a company that sells products for kidney disease patients. In such an instance one is reminded of the famous quote attributed to Pulitzer Prize–winning writer and activist Upton Sinclair: 'It is difficult to get a man to understand something when his salary depends on his not understanding it.'

Once exposed, however, Furnival demonstrated little remorse, announcing that his February 2014 resignation was given with the knowledge that neither he nor his wife had done anything wrong and that his conscience was clear. One might wonder what Dr Margaret Chan would make of such a curiously un-self-aware defence.

Incidentally, the National Health Star Ratings scheme ultimately came under fire virtually as soon as it was launched. Food items such as butter or Greek yoghurt have been given half a star due to their saturated-fat content, while omega-6-filled processed foods get a free ride due to their polyunsaturated status. Manufacturers have boosted their star rating by adding an additional healthier product to the combination. For example, Milo on its own is given a 1.5 but when skim milk is added it claims a 4.5-star rating. Some sugary breakfast cereals feature a 3.5-star rating on the side of the box that appears to be the rating but is in fact part of an 'explanatory rating', while the lower rating the product was actually given can be found on the front of the box – not the usual place people look for consumer information.

Another disturbing arrangement occurred when the Australian Heart Foundation accepted AU$300,000 from McDonald's to put its 'Tick' on several of its foods, including fried foods. It also allowed Pizza Cutters to include the Tick on its pizzas. Even Four'N Twenty meat pies and an Ingham's turkey schnitzel at one point or another carried the Tick. While the Australian Heart Foundation claimed its credibility was intact, a supermarket shelf review of many of the products listed as heart-friendly were heavily processed and would not fit the criteria of what many would consider health-promoting. After a 2014 social media campaign and petition, the Heart Foundation pledged to consider the feedback within the Tick review process conducted by 'external experts with public health, nutrition, business and food industry credentials'. By the end of

2015, the Heart Foundation finally recognised officially that the Tick was past its use-by date and consigned it to the annals of history. The question remains, however, would this have happened without public pressure?

Possibly the most explosive case of corporate patronage of prominent academics came to light in 2015. Back in 2012, Rhona S. Applebaum, Coca-Cola's chief food scientist, spoke at a food industry conference. She outlined the drink maker's strategy of nurturing relationships with top scientists in an effort to balance the narrative on the role of sugary drinks in the health crisis. To this end, Coca-Cola had spent US$1.5 million supporting a not-for-profit group called Global Energy Balance Network, whose president was notable obesity researcher Professor James O. Hill. The University of Colorado medical school where Professor Hill works as a researcher received US$1 million of the Coca-Cola money as a grant.

In one of a damning series of emails made public in 2015 by Associated Press, Professor Hill offered to run a large and expensive 'game changer' study that would provide a strong justification for 'why a company selling sugar water SHOULD focus on promoting physical activity'. Hill also admitted in the emails that he wanted to work with the drinks company to help manage its image problem. While in response to the leaks Coca-Cola trotted out the standard industry line that despite its financial contribution, it had no influence over the activities of the group, further reports showed that Applebaum and Coca-Cola executives not only helped pick the group's management but design its website and develop its mission statement. Applebaum stepped down from the drinks company in late 2015.

As the leaders of the dietetics and public-health world continue to display behaviour like this, routinely availing themselves of industry money and continuing on their long-established path of failing to arrest a painfully obvious public-health crisis, we have to ask whether they are capable of doing their job. But what if they *are* doing their job but it just doesn't align with public expectation? In a scientific statement regarding processed foods released by the American Society for Nutrition, a list of 'stakeholder' responsibilities proved quite illuminating on this issue. It turns out that stakeholders in the processed-food industry are many (far more than one might realise) and diverse. And they all have different jobs to do. For example, healthcare professionals can promote the healthy uses of processed food, incorporate healthy processed foods into educational opportunities and create partnerships with the food industry to help patients.

Maybe that explains why, during my time as a dialysis patient, I was taught by a specialist kidney dietitian how to manage my fluid intake using an educational poster covered in sugary drinks manufactured by the processed-food industry. Even Red Bull was on the poster. The poster was 'supported' by a pharmaceutical company. Perhaps worse, however, was being given a brochure 'supported' by a kidney peak organisation advising me to replace protein (evidently bad for hurt kidneys) with 'free foods' or high-energy foods upon which there was no restriction. Examples listed in order included sugar/glucose, jam/honey/marmalade, syrups/toppings/icings, ice blocks, soft drinks/cordials, boiled lollies/jelly beans/similar lollies, cornflower/sago/tapioca/arrowroot, poly- and monounsaturated margarines, oils and salad dressings. The tagline of the brochure said, 'You'll be the only person on the block on a jelly bean diet'.

Hmmmm. Such experiences were so disheartening during my time on dialysis. It's like a punch in the stomach to realise that for even the sickest of hospital patients, nothing is sacred.

The revolving doors between industry, government and academia, the funding of diet and health institutions by food and drug companies, and the constant stream of confusing media messages from organisations that purport to serve public health all leave consumers with no real option but to find what works best for them. This is where the micropowers come in. As Margaret Chan points out, we must push back on the food industry's efforts to shape the public-health policies that effect its products, because when it does, the most effective control measures are downplayed or excluded. 'This,' cautions Chan, 'is well documented, and dangerous.'

9

The rise and rise of the wellness industry

Fed-up consumers everywhere are now demanding more alternatives to traditional health care, as a result of the perfect storm created by rising consumer concern about growing levels of obesity and chronic disease; the blatant inability of our health agencies and various experts to stem the problem; a documented rise in allergies, intolerances and autoimmunity; revelations surrounding our diet's vital role in the health of our microbiome and our genome; and our rapidly growing disillusionment with perceived 'captured agencies'. Like Weston Price's indigenous research subjects, many of us now want to get off the reservation. We want a return to health, not just for ourselves, but for our children and the generations still to come. And one thing is clear: we will not get a different result by doing the same thing or listening to the same people who helped us into the current chronic-disease mess.

Over the last few years, the concept of 'wellness' has entered our lexicon, and a new breed of young and not-so-young 'health and wellness warriors' have stepped into the arena, ready to lead the way forward. Pilates, massage, yoga and reflexology centres have proliferated on trendy retail strips. Bearded hipsters have been spotted peddling around inner-city suburbs downing blended greens in mason jars. Paleo cafés offering fresh, organic and 'free-from' options are packing in the unabashedly health-conscious crowds. About Life, the health and wellness-oriented combined supermarket and café chain that started in Sydney, opened in Melbourne in 2016. In 2015, Melbourne's first 'allergen-free' café opened – the brainchild of a young couple affected by food intolerance and desperate for somewhere safe to eat out. Necessity really is the mother of invention.

Wellness has been dismissed by sceptics as a fad, but the sheer numbers of people embracing it and the dollars being spent in pursuit of it would suggest it's anything but. What sceptics don't appear to grasp is the fact that consumers in 2017 are educated, informed, discerning, integrity and truth-seeking, financially selective, and media and technology savvy. They exist in an age of information, with access to a diversity of news, views, conversational media and online communities. No longer content to take their cue from the traditional press, consumers are looking for new health authorities that deliver information and solutions relevant to their particular health needs. Wellness has well and truly gone mainstream.

The wellness movement represents a 'recalibration' or 'ratcheting-up' of the human body and the human spirit to form a better fit with the world in which we now find ourselves. Just as

Weston Price's indigenous groups were scarcely able to survive the fatal mismatch between their highly tuned ancestral genes and the blunt impact of sugar and wheat, we too appear to have stumbled into a world to which we are struggling to adapt, physically and psychologically. The chronic-disease epidemic is a potent reminder that there is little point creating a 'modern world' if we are unable to survive its impact.

Antifragility

The term 'antifragile' was coined by Nassim Nicholas Taleb, ex-trader and current distinguished professor of risk engineering at New York University's School of Engineering, in his 2012 book *Antifragile: Things That Gain From Disorder*. Taleb argues that humans and systems appear to thrive under conditions that throw up environmental stressors such as randomness and volatility – provided they engage in 'antifragile tinkering' that enables adaptation to the environment. The 'antifragile' takes stressors as information and responds accordingly. The 'antifragile' is curious, takes risks, 'fails small' and 'fails fast'. Antifragility is 'part of our ancestral behaviour, our biological apparatus, and a ubiquitous property of every system that has survived'. If the bureaucrat is fragile, the entrepreneur is antifragile. If industry is fragile, the artisan is antifragile. If post-traumatic stress is fragile, post-traumatic growth is antifragile. 'Antifragility is *beyond* resilience or robustness. The resilient resists shocks and stays the same, the antifragile gets better' (my italics).

According to Taleb, the fragile or 'fragilista' does not respond well to volatility, randomness, disorder, errors or environmental stressors, and appears to remain rigid in response to chaos. Preferring to attempt to control the environment rather than adapt to it, the fragile are ultimately breakable and, worse, inflict fragility on others. For example:

- The medical fragilista ignores the natural ability of our bodies to heal themselves of many health conditions, instead intervening with medications that could have severe side effects.
- The policy fragilista behaves as a social planner who intervenes in economic or health systems in an attempt to fix them, but ultimately makes everything worse.
- The psychiatric fragilista seeks to medicate children in an attempt to improve them, but in many cases damages them further while failing to solve underlying problems.
- The 'soccer-mum fragilista' oversees the most minute details of their children's life, to the point where the child lacks much-needed resilience in adulthood.
- The financial fragilista applies risk models to the banking system, corrupting and ultimately destroying it.
- The military fragilista intervenes in complex systems, creating social and political turmoil that result in war and upheaval in previously peaceful countries.

If mass medicine is fragile (and inflicts fragility on others), one might argue that the collective shift toward wellness is antifragile. If the top-down food-pyramid-style diet is fragile, nutrigenomics – which builds a diet based around the effects of diet on an individual's genetic profile – is antifragile. Taleb surmises in the book that ultimately only the antifragile survive. Today's health consumers are learning that wellness-based tinkering may in fact be the key not just to surviving in today's world, but to thriving. Mass is out, customised is in.

Further supporting this idea is the concept of 'previving', which was coined by trends forecaster Martin Raymond. Previving describes the shift towards more people embracing personal health and wellness strategies and behaviours designed to *prevent* them becoming ill. In addition to preventing illness, I would add that people are engaging in health and wellness behaviours in order to better *survive* a past or current health crisis. For many people a minor or major health scare is enough to make them rethink past behaviours – such as poor eating habits, lack of exercise, smoking, low awareness of how diet and behaviour lead to sickness, a high-stress lifestyle, bad relationships or drug and alcohol abuse – and commit to a better way forward in the future.

I remember, during a particular set of hospital visits, spending time with a nurse who had worked with cancer patients for decades. She told me about the many young people she had looked after during their cancer treatments and how, when they returned for check-ups months or years later, the majority of them had committed to much healthier diets and lifestyles than they had practised before, and many were almost sheepish about how little attention they had previously paid to their health.

The wellness movement

If the 'traditional media' representations of the wellness movement are anything to go by, one could be forgiven for believing it to be a disorganised gaggle of fringe dwellers peddling 'unscientific quackery'. The reality is somewhat different, which is why traditional health authorities and pharmaceutical companies are worried. According to research by the agency SRI International, the global Spa and Wellness industry was by 2013 worth a staggering US$3.4 trillion annually, almost three and a half times the value of the global pharmaceutical market. This industry cluster comprises four sectors:

- wellness lifestyle products and services (US$2806 billion)
- wellness tourism (US$494 billion)
- spa industry (US$94 billion)
- thermal/mineral springs (US$50 billion).

The 'wellness lifestyle' industry grew by 62 per cent between 2010 and 2013, driven by our growing desire to look and feel good, maintain our health and prevent illness. The growth of the global pharmaceutical industry, by contrast, has been relatively flat for several years, and its projected 2015–18 growth rate is only 2.1 per cent in advanced economies and 6 per cent in emerging markets. It's somewhat ironic that greater financial growth can be achieved in helping people make the shift towards health and wellness, than by selling them drugs that keep them trapped inside the hamster wheel of chronic disease. Corporate wellness has also cemented itself as a worthwhile 'people' investment, as business increasingly learns that the cost of keeping employees well (and productive) is infinitely lower than paying for them when they are sick, absent and unproductive. A comprehensive report on corporate wellness published by RAND Corporation in 2013 revealed that employee participation in a workplace wellness program is associated with a trend towards lower healthcare costs and decreasing healthcare use.

The obvious financial rewards associated with wellness will continue to attract interest and financial investment from a new breed of entrepreneurs drawn to the 'doing well by doing good' business model. Excited by the idea of generating wealth by bringing health and happiness to people's lives (and our planet) via authentic, clean, natural, environmentally sustainable products and services in addition to highly creative bespoke health solutions, the wellness entrepreneur will focus on responding to consumer demand for 'anytime, anyplace' health.

The wellness lifestyle industries can themselves be broken down into seven categories:

1. healthy eating/nutrition and weight loss (US$574 billion)
2. complementary and alternative medicine (US$187 billion)
3. preventative/personalised health (US$433 billion)
4. fitness and mind–body (US$446 billion)
5. beauty and anti-ageing (US$1026 billion)
6. workplace wellness (US$41 billion)
7. wellness lifestyle real estate (US$100 billion).

The combined global healthy eating/nutrition and weight loss, and preventative/personalised health market sectors are worth just over US$1 trillion, indicating that consumers are making food choices with health and disease prevention in mind. According to a survey by Palo Alto's Institute for the Future, more than half of adults (52 per cent) believe that good nutrition prevents most chronic diseases; 58 per cent believe that good nutrition eliminates the need for most prescription drugs; and 70 per cent believe that good nutrition delays the onset of most chronic diseases.

As more people begin to place a high value upon health, they will enter the market looking for personalised, modifiable and sustainable end-to-end health solutions that fit their lifestyle, rather than depend solely on medications and their possible side effects. This increased awareness and understanding of the intimate connection between food and disease prevention and management is clearly driving increased growth in this sector. There are several drivers and enablers of the movement towards wellness with the ultimate goal of achieving antifragility within our built world, the most salient being:

- the pervasiveness of social networking
- rapidly advancing technological innovation
- rising consumer demands for clean, sustainable solutions
- high expectations concerning authenticity and trust.

Social networking

In 2007, the Institute for the Future examined the emergence of a new contributor to the health and healthcare conversation – the biocitizen. The concept of the biocitizen describes people who form online networks based on shared health values or medical conditions. These networks may be patient groups such as those suffering diabetes or breast cancer; specific diet groups such as vegan or low-carb; or groups involved in health-lobbying movements such as those pushing for GMO labelling in the United States or sugar taxes.

Under the traditional model of health, information has been developed and packaged by 'experts' and 'authorities' – such as disease or organ foundations, dietetics experts, doctors, corporations and the media – in a top-down, one-way approach. For years, consumers have been conditioned into a passive relationship, exemplified by the standard food-pyramid diet and the patriarchal medical model, where everything has been decided for them and where questioning the 'wisdom of experts' is unheard of. This model appeared to be acceptable to the 'silent generation' and even many baby boomers, but the emerging biocitizen refuses to consume such dictates passively, preferring to participate actively in creating bottom-up media content that reflects the desire for participatory and collaborative approaches to health management. Such user-generated or conversational media includes health blogs, Wikipedia entries, discussion forums, video and audio files, podcasts, social media pages and medical-data-aggregation sites such as GreenMedInfo.

As interconnected members of the global village, biocitizens can locate and disseminate information such as the latest medical literature on heart disease or autoimmunity, circumventing and even 'pushing back' against the traditional filtering health organisations in their search for knowledge, insight, truth and trust. They share information on health products, services, and local vegan or Paleo cafés. They rate the allergen-free status of restaurants, airlines and hotels; the effectiveness of cancer doctors; and the cleanliness of hospitals. They openly discuss the side effects of medications and expose underhand tactics used by food corporations to create anti-consumer laws – naming, shaming and ultimately eroding public trust in valuable corporate brands. They influence purchasing decisions and how products are used, providing real-life and even real-time feedback about their experience with Paleo diets, weight-loss shakes or supplements.

Biocitizens have created a rapidly growing 'collective intelligence' – the convergence of combined knowledge and shared experience of large groups of people with a common interest or goal. In short, biocitizens are not looking for permission – they are busy rewriting the rules of engagement. While traditional health authorities outwardly dismiss biocitizens as neurotic 'Dr Google types', they inwardly worry about the battle for relevancy in which they are unwittingly and unwillingly engaged and for which they are seemingly ill prepared.

Websites

Social networking provides many opportunities for 'anytime, anywhere' health. Today, many of the most popular weight-loss websites offer not just diet advice and recipes but videos of health experts and exercise techniques, and dynamic forums where dieters can connect with and support others with similar goals or even join a weight-loss 'team'. Websites such as MindBodyGreen enable people to undertake online courses led by experts in health, wellness and movement at their own leisure and streamed via their tablet, home computer or smartphone. According to the global internet rankings site Alexa, the website Gluten-Free Girl is one of the top-ranked nutrition websites in the world, ahead of Nutrition.gov, America's federal nutrition guide. Gluten-Free Girl offers cooking videos, gluten-free recipes, baking classes, Instagram updates, book tour 'meet and greets', daily blog posts and gluten-related Q&A. Who needs a dietitian when you have Gluten-Free Girl?

YouTube

YouTube, the million-channel network of the people, today features many videos of doctors and medical researchers talking about their discoveries. Paediatric endocrinologist Professor Robert Lustig's lecture at the University of California titled 'Sugar: the bitter truth' went viral and has now been seen by more than 6 million people, an audience size considered unthinkable only a few years ago for what was in fact a routine university lecture. Dr Terry Wahl's talk on recovering from severe symptoms of multiple sclerosis has been watched more than 2 million times. American surgeon and former McKinsey consultant Dr Peter Attia, in his TED Talk titled 'What if we're wrong about diabetes?', details his recovery from metabolic syndrome and insulin resistance by turning his back on the carbohydrate-heavy food pyramid, and his current work in helping to end the diabetes epidemic. His emotional talk, where he confesses to having wrongly judged obese patients for their 'self-inflicted' diabetes, has been viewed thousands of times.

Podcasts

Wellness podcasts such as the 'Rich Roll Podcast', Jimmy Moore's long-running 'Livin' La Vida Low-Carb' show and 'Underground Wellness' are popular thanks to their high-quality guests and interesting topics. The year 2013 saw the world's first online 'Gluten Summit', which featured more than 30 interviews with medical experts such as Drs Michael Marsh (creator of the Marsh system used by gastroenterologists in diagnosing coeliac disease), Umberto Volta, Alessio Fasano, Yehuda Shoenfeld and Aristo Vojdani – all considered world leaders in their respective fields. The summit was open to the public, with transcripts and presentation materials available to purchase at a very affordable price. Other popular online summits, covering such topics as depression, thyroid disease, autoimmunity, heart disease, wellness and diabetes, have given global audiences the opportunity to hear from some of the world's top medical experts, thought leaders and entrepreneurs in these fields. Health summits enable biocitizens to learn more about their own health conditions by connecting directly with independent experts who are offering the latest scientific insights and practical health solutions.

Technological innovation

As biocitizens shift away from seeing health as the sole responsibility of a doctor to a more self-managed approach, they are increasingly seeking technological solutions that enable deeper insight into their personal health status.

The Quantified Self movement

The Quantified Self or Personal Informatics movement that has emerged in recent years is synonymous with the notion of personalised and participatory health. The Quantified Self community is global and growing rapidly. In 2015, it held its sixth annual conference in San Francisco, which focused on wearable devices and apps that provide 'intimate and direct feedback about yourself, from how you sleep, eat, and exercise, to what triggers fear and joy'. While some of the 2015 presentations such as 'Track your baby for fun' or 'Track your sneezes' may appear to be a disturbing or puzzling use of technology, other uses included alcohol-consumption tracking, diet tracking for cancer support, anticoagulation-therapy tracking, sleep tracking and gut-bacteria tracking, in addition to the newly popularised movement, exercise and fitness tracking technologies. Such technologies allow biocitizens to obtain quantitative and qualitative baseline and variability data points for various-health related issues and contributing behaviours, allowing them to see the effects of various inputs over specific time frames.

Elite athletes are now using Quantified Self technologies to remarkable effect. The 2015 documentary *Personal Gold: An Underdog Story* tells of a group of down-and-out female cyclists who undertook a Quantified Self 'data not doping' experiment in their quest to compete in the London Olympics, and subsequently won a silver medal in the team pursuit event. One of the key technologies used by the team was InsideTracker, a personalised home blood-testing kit that reveals the status of twenty biomarkers considered most essential to overall wellbeing and athletic performance. It's available worldwide, which means that users anywhere may undergo blood analysis and obtain customised nutrition, supplements, lifestyle and exercise regimens most suitable to their unique biochemistry.

Many biocitizens are interested in wearable technologies that track physical activity, such as Fitbit, Slimband, Apple Watch, Jawbone UP and Misfit Wearables; or track sleep, such as Zeo, Beddit and WakeMate; along with app-based technologies that track diet, weight and fertility cycles. While some may argue that these technologies may lead to micromanaging daily behaviours and consequently new forms of neurosis, used properly, they enable users not just to gain an insight into their behaviours but to see first hand how a commitment to behavioural change can lead to positive long-term results.

Online studies and crowd-sourcing

Biocitizens are increasingly turning to participatory online health studies. Some sign up to PatientsLikeMe, a 350,000-member website covering 2500 health conditions and 28 million disease-related data points. It seeks to enable people to compare their treatments, experiences and symptoms with others in similar situations and to benefit from treatment breakthroughs. In 2015, PatientsLikeMe announced a research collaboration agreement with the FDA to determine how patient-reported data could give new insights into drug safety. The website gives patients with specific diseases a collective voice in the wilderness. It enables them to submit ideas and data that will help medical researchers better understand and treat diseases, and potentially expedite the reporting of drug-safety and side-effect information to authorities.

Biocitizens who are part of a specific patient community can now crowd-fund research studies that may benefit them directly. Paleo chef Pete Evans gave a shout-out on his Facebook page in 2014 for a group of American researchers seeking crowd-funding to study the effects of the Paleo diet on women with PCOS. Genomera is an internet-based organisation that crowd-sources genomic and phenotypic information it then analyses free of charge. While still a small organisation, it represents the emerging trend toward 'citizen science', where ordinary people can participate in research specific to their interests. Biocitizens will increasingly be able to target and connect with scientific researchers around the world, offering them non-traditional funding sources and genomic data in exchange for science-based insights into various health conditions, their causes and how they may be better managed.

Gene testing

At the time of writing, consumer genomics company 23andMe offered a US$149 'loss-leader' genetic test kit that maps customers' genomes and gives them ancestry information. The company caused some controversy after it admitted to sharing consumer data with pharmaceutical companies and the revelation of its partial funding by tech giant Google. In 2013, the FDA barred 23andMe from issuing genetics-based health reports to customers, and the company can now only offer one genetic test, for Bloom syndrome. The company has since confirmed it will move into drug development. This may not sit well with some biocitizens, who express a preference for obtaining 'actionable' personal information aligned with wellness and prevention rather than more medications.

One of the ways biocitizens are using genetic data to acquire personally actionable 'wellness' information is by firstly obtaining their raw data via a genetic test from a company such as 23andme and uploading it to an online genetic analysis tool such as Promethease for a small fee. Promethease is a freeware computer program developed by SNPedia, a wiki-based bioinformatics website drawing on a database of more than 73,000 SNPs that may be associated with disease risk. Using this information, biocitizens can identify specific markers that can be modified by diet and lifestyle changes to lower the risk of developing in the short or long term a health problem to which they are predisposed.

One of the most common SNPs biocitizens are on the lookout for are those associated with the gene coding for an enzyme called methylene-tetrahydrofolate reductase (MTHFR) on chromosome 1. MTHFR is involved in converting folate (vitamin B9, from eggs and green leafy vegetables) into its active form, 5-methyltetrahydrofolate.

In this form, folate is involved in the conversion of the amino acid homocysteine to another amino acid, methionine. A fault or mutation in the MTHFR gene can cause a toxic build-up of homocysteine in the blood, which has been associated with a number of health conditions, such as coronary artery disease, chronic fatigue, multiple sclerosis, infertility, addictions and mental health issues among others.

Bioinformaticist Raymond McCauley obtained his raw genetic data from 23andMe and, after learning about his genetic predispositions to diabetes, obesity and cardiovascular problems, made a concerted effort to lose weight. McCauley's data also revealed that he had a 30 per cent lifetime risk of age-related macular degeneration, a condition linked to folate and vitamin B12 deficiency and high homocysteine levels.

McCauley teamed up with a group of people to investigate whether the MTHFR gene could respond to vitamin supplementation and lower their blood homocysteine levels. The experiment involved two weeks of no supplementation followed by a period in which the group took supermarket multivitamins. In these, the folate is in the form of folic acid, which requires an extra biochemical step in the human body to become active. The group then switched to taking the more active L-methylfolate form, and then a period of combining this with the multivitamins, followed by a period of no supplementation. Blood samples were taken during each of the phases to measure homocysteine levels. In four of the participants, homocysteine levels dropped by almost one-third, regardless of the type of vitamin supplement used. For McCauley (who had the highest MTHFR risk) the supermarket multivitamins *raised* homocysteine levels, while L-methylfolate was the only supplement that lowered them. He now takes L-methylfolate regularly.

This exercise in nutrigenomics, normally restricted to scientists with an understanding of genetics and nutrition, will one day become commonplace. Biocitizens will routinely investigate and manage their own nutrigenomic profile in conjunction with a doctor or genetics expert rather than take standardised advice from a dietitian or other health authority.

Self-experimentation

Many biocitizens care little for scientific findings, preferring their own direct experience with a diet, product or behavioural change, and reaching their own conclusion as to its effectiveness. For example, if a biocitizen decides to remove gluten, soy and sugar from their diet or undertake CrossFit classes, then experiences rapid health improvements as a result, they will not revert to behaviours that didn't serve them just because traditional health authorities, who are working from population-level information, tell them to. Biocitizens are often interested in achieving a health goal or solving a health problem (where practicable) through self-experimentation and iteration of various interventions, known as 'learning arcs', until they achieve the desirable end point.

For example, a biocitizen with sleep problems may work their way through several interventions, including removal of stimulants before bed, removal of technological devices from bedrooms, a 20-minute pre-sleep relaxation process or even altering the position of their bed, to determine the best solution. A doctor may recommend potentially addictive sleeping medication for the same issue, based upon population data that does not take individual biochemistry, environment or personal circumstances into consideration.

'Clean' values and sustainable solutions

As people begin to value their health more, they will make increasing demands on the online and traditional retail marketplace to provide them with specific 'solutions'. The US online retailer Thrive Market, for example, enables customers to 'shop by their values', organising food products according to organic, GMO-free, Paleo, gluten-free, raw, vegan or 'moms' principles. This online shopping club is publicly endorsed by some of the most prominent names in the wellness industry, including personal trainer Jillian Michaels. In a classic case of 'doing well by doing good', Thrive Market is using technology to bring quality foods to all Americans, regardless of income or location.

According to global research conducted by Nielsen, today's consumers are going 'back to basics' in their food preferences – rating 'fresh', 'natural' and 'unprocessed' as desirable attributes for food purchases. With GMO-labelling efforts gaining momentum globally, it's no surprise that 43 per cent of respondents see GMO labelling as an important factor in purchase decisions. This may result in more food producers opting for voluntary 'GMO-free' labels to entice consumers, given consumers value GMO-free foods even more highly than they do organics.

WHAT ARE GMO FOODS?

In the context of food, genetically modified organisms are generally plants in which the DNA has been scientifically altered in some way, by splicing in a gene (breaking and inserting) from another

---

organism. This might be, for example, a gene transferred from the bacterium *Bacillus thuringiensis* (which is commonly used in organic biological control) to corn to make the corn resistant to insect pests.

Australia has GMO-labelling laws by which foods produced from GMOs must be labelled as 'genetically modified' when they still contain the modified DNA after processing. Where the GMO is highly refined to the extent that there is none of the modified DNA in the final product, such as soybean oil for example, the product need not be labelled as genetically modified.

The global appetite for organic products has increased five-fold since 1999, indicating the consumer desire for pesticide- and herbicide-free foods. Australia has the world's largest supply of organic agricultural land, with 17.2 million hectares out of 43.1 million hectares globally, and is well positioned to become the organic capital of the world. Global sales of organic foods recently stood at US$72 billion, with 90 per cent of the demand coming from the United States and Europe. Retail sales for organic products in Australia during 2013 totalled US$1.1 billion, while American sales totalled US$26.7 billion.

According to the Nielsen research, more than 60 per cent of respondents are cutting down on sugar and fats, while 57 per cent are eating more natural and fresh foods. Around 46 per cent of North American respondents are eating fewer processed foods. In addition, 35 per cent of respondents placed significant importance on sustainably sourced ingredients, and a further 26 per cent rated local-grown ingredients as very important.

The rapidly rising popularity of the farmers' market, slow food and paddock-to-plate movements reflect the consumer interest in where our food comes from, who is growing it and under what conditions. Health-conscious consumers are also increasingly concerned about food safety in the light of several major food scares in recent years, and are more aware of the importance of 'country of origin' labelling.

During a recent frozen berries scare in Australia, I asked a local berry farmer why the farmers did not produce enough berries for Australian consumers, given the safety issues of foreign foods. The farmer replied that Australian farmers grew more than enough for the Australian people but due to trade deals, made more money sending the berries to overseas buyers. The farmer was staggered that as an Australian farmer he was growing berries according to very strict safety standards for people living in another country, while the health of his local community and fellow Australians was put at risk by consuming berries grown under much lower safety standards. The farmers' market movement is the best way to avoid these safety blunders, as consumers deal with the farmer directly. Another way is growing your own.

Authenticity and trust

Today's food consumers are more discerning than ever, and the issue of 'food trust' has become a top priority for many health-conscious citizens, who are increasingly keen to know more about not just products and their ingredients but the corporate behaviours of manufacturers and retailers alike. Bottom-up vigilance from consumers means businesses are increasingly being held accountable for breaches of trust, and some even publicly named and shamed for engaging in behaviours such as environmental damage, excessive chemical use, exploitation of workers, contribution to the obesity epidemic, treatment of women and children, land grabs and slave labour.

Agricultural chemical company Monsanto has been on the receiving end of consumer rage for several years due to its gene-patenting technologies, which have led to accusations of monopolising vital aspects of the food supply; continuing to sell its top-selling herbicide Roundup (which contains glyphosate, a product that has been listed as 'probably carcinogenic' by the International Agency Research on Cancer, and whose use has increased by 400 per cent in the last twenty years in the United Kingdom alone); government lobbying to minimise business regulation with relation to GMO foods; and poor treatment of subsistence farmers in India, leading to suicides. Growing consumer awareness of Monsanto's practices has led to the March Against Monsanto, now held around the world every year.

Organisations that consistently fail to respond to food-trust issues will increasingly find themselves on the outer with health-conscious consumers, who now form a large part of the market. This situation has the potential to translate into billions of dollars in lost sales for manufacturers and retailers alike. Successful food businesses of the future will see the value in pursuing comprehensive food-trust practices to help pilot their valuable brands through increasingly choppy waters.

Whether they call themselves consumers, biocitizens or quantified selfers, those interested in happier and healthier lives are no longer afraid to vote with their feet and their wallets in their quest for authentic and trusted suppliers of not just foods but wellness products and services. If a supplement doesn't work, they won't buy it; if a Paleo diet doesn't make them feel better, they won't follow it; if a restaurant can't offer them a gluten-free meal option, they won't visit again; if supermarkets can't provide clearly labelled nutritionally customised food solutions, they will find a specialty retailer that will. Brand loyalty (indeed any type of loyalty) has become a rare bird in a very bustling marketplace offering a multitude of options and inputs for our quest for antifragility.

By allocating discretionary income to wellness offerings such as Paleo cookbooks or gluten-free foods, consumers are anticipating something in return. They are an increasingly tough crowd to please, and they are firmly in the driver's seat. They control the exchange, and if you want their dollar, you had better be relevant. Commenting on the 2015 closures of hundreds of McDonald's restaurants across the United States, Japan and China, Mike Donahue, former chief of communications for McDonald's and cofounder of rapidly growing healthy-options restaurant chain LYFE Kitchen, said, 'the only thing that stops growth is relevancy to the customer'. Indeed, while McDonald's restaurants have been closing, chains like Chipotle Mexican Grill that market themselves as clean, healthy or 100 per cent GMO-free have been experiencing extraordinary growth. The message is simple: if McDonald's can't adjust to consumer concerns about food, the people will simply take their wallets and go elsewhere.

Given the rapid and extraordinary growth of the wellness market, it's of little surprise to find the pharmaceutical industry beginning to circle. Sluggish growth in mainstay businesses has forced the industry to move into uncharted but lucrative waters. In 2009, drug giant Pfizer acquired supplement manufacturer Centrum through its Wyeth takeover deal and partially attributed double-digit sales of its consumer health products in its fourth quarter 2012 to 'strong growth' of Centrum. In 2011, Pfizer bought Ferrosan Consumer Health, a Danish supplements company, and Alacer Corp, a manufacturer of powdered vitamin drinks. Paul Surman, president of Pfizer's consumer division, acknowledged that 'consumers are taking increasing personal responsibility for their own health and wellness ... Vitamins and dietary supplements play an important and direct role in this.' Reckitt Benckiser has also identified supplements as an area for growth, acquiring Airborne and outbidding rival Bayer for Schiff Nutrition for US$1.4 billion in 2012. Procter & Gamble acquired supplements maker New Chapter, and Johnson & Johnson's McNeil Nutritionals sells dietary supplements and lactose-free milk products.

In 2015, Australian vitamin manufacturer Swisse was sold to Hong Kong–listed company Biostime International Holdings for AU$1.67 billion, beating Hony Capital and Shanghai Pharma to seal the deal. The share price of well-known Australian vitamin brand Blackmores rocketed from AU$31 per share to more than AU$200 in the space of one year due to explosive demand for its 'clean and green' products from desperate consumers in China. In terms of share price, Blackmores has outperformed traditional blue-chip companies such as Cochlear, CSL, Macquarie Bank and the Commonwealth Bank. The listed Australian organic company Bellamy's Organic has had trouble meeting demand for its organic baby formula from both local and Chinese consumers. The call for clean products from Asian consumers demonstrates a certain level of fear and concern regarding the quality of their own food supplies. Bellamy's listed at AU$1.00 per share in August 2014 before surging 1225 per cent to AU$13.25 in December 2015.

The food industry has also stepped up its interest in wellness, with Nestlé Health Science investing US$65 million in Seres Health, a start-up that focuses on restoring the microbiome. In addition, Nestlé Health Science acquired Prometheus Laboratories, a firm that creates personalised therapies for bowel-based diseases. It has also partnered with venture capital to help advance start-ups in the nutritional therapy field. Greg Behar, chief executive of Nestlé Health Science noted that in specific diseases, nutrition plays an important role, and therapeutic nutrition thus presents a growth opportunity.

Wellness and government

So big is the wellness industry expected to grow that Susie Ellis, chair and CEO of the Global Wellness Institute, insists that governments around the world must seriously consider the possibility of introducing a national Ministry of Wellness to help repair their broken healthcare systems. Rather than relying on overburdened hospitals to operate as 'fix-it shops' focused on treating symptoms, the idea would be to create a ministry that focuses solely on preventative care.

Some governments have already taken steps in this direction: Canadian provinces Alberta and Nova Scotia, and tiny Caribbean nation Saint Vincent and the Grenadines have all set up Ministries for Health and Wellness. In 2014, India's prime minister, Narendra Modi, appointed India's first Minister for Ayurveda, Yoga, Naturopathy, Unani, Siddha and Homeopathy (AYUSH Minister), Shripad Yesso Naik. 'We will do whatever it takes to make India a healthy India in the days ahead,' said Naik. Prime Minister Modi has also called for an international yoga day.

Wellness is an industry that, to borrow another term from Nassim Taleb, is only 'half-invented' and thus has a tremendous amount of growth yet to come. Turning around the health of millions of people is an enormous job that requires easy-to-access education and health-management solutions. One of the key areas that will experience this growth is the food system, as shopping for food will take on greater significance as part of the 'anytime, anyplace' health model. Helping people in all walks to engage in 'antifragile tinkering' will become big business, as the patient model of care gives way to the consumer model – and ultimately the biocitizen model – of personalised health management.

10

Mother Nature obeyed

If we now have a better understanding of what renders people susceptible to sickness and we know that one diet does not fit all, then what *does* make people healthy? What *are* the common denominators of health and wellness? Dr Weston Price went in search of the answer to this question in 1931. Not only did he uncover the answer, but he begged us to avail ourselves of the accumulated wisdom of the generations of fit, strong, healthy and happy people that preceded us. He did so not just so that we could secure the knowledge for ourselves, but so that we could pass on this extraordinary and most valuable inheritance to those generations not yet born, and in the process secure our survival as a species.

The secret discovered by Dr Price is simple, and he summed it up in perhaps his most famous quote: 'Life in all its fullness is this Mother Nature obeyed.'

In an era when a near dietary dictatorship prevails and the act of cutting out a food group without medical justification will potentially earn you a diagnosis of a mental illness such as 'orthorexia', it's refreshingly noteworthy that Price's information was not distilled from research papers by prestigious universities and industry-funded nutrition institutes (and nutritionists!), but by thousands – and in some cases millions – of years of human history. The tribal wisdom presented by Dr Price is underpinned by a virtuous cycle of continuous adaptation. This is achieved through a constant process of elegant refinement, its divinely inspired goal to provide humanity with a physical form capable of surviving and indeed thriving in its environment, however hostile conditions may become.

Perhaps Dr Price's greatest lesson for us is the realisation that throughout history, humans have been capable of drawing sustenance from a broad range of natural foods that were freely available within their local environments. They had no need of dietary advice from 'experts', as both their diet and secrets to healthy living were handed down to them by their elders. While today's elders pass on assets and trinkets, Dr Price's indigenous elders passed on the most important inheritance we can ever receive – the tried and tested keys to survival for both the individual and the community.

So what were those secrets and how can we adapt them to today's modern world? We can boil them down into four main categories:

1. eating traditional, nutrient-dense foods
2. using traditional food preparation, preservation and storage methods
3. protecting the health of future generations
4. living a traditional lifestyle.

Eating traditional, nutrient-dense whole foods

1. **Whole foods were eaten to avoid the loss of vitamins, minerals, fibre and enzymes.** Processing whole foods renders them nutritionally void and often involves the use of chemicals, which adds to our chemical burden.

   Many whole foods are available to us today, such as organically and locally grown GMO-free vegetables, fruits, animal proteins, fats, nuts, seeds, and soaked/fermented or sprouted grains and legumes. These are easy to obtain from farmers' markets, specialty stores, online organic retailers and in the organic food sections of major supermarket chains.

   There is also an abundance of cookery books boasting hundreds of recipes and cooking hints, in addition to online communities to aid us in creating new and interesting meals at home. Favourite recipes can be shared and, with today's technology, can be turned into a book, which can be given as a gift to younger generations.

   I personally stick to organic foods whenever I can (mostly to avoid farm chemicals), and I buy from farmers' markets, organic shops or grow my own in the back garden. I buy high-quality free-range, grass-fed meat from a particular farmer I have known for a long time. His farm is sustainable, he treats the animals humanely and he does not use hormones, grains, antibiotics or animal feeds with GMOs. As meat is part of the diet in our house, we choose to spend our money with a farmer who shares our ethos.

2. **Fats were never the enemy.** In fact, they provided essential energy and nutrition to those hardy individuals with whom Price came into contact. Sources we can draw upon include butter from organic, grass-fed cows; avocado; coconut and olive oil; animal meat and organs, including seafood; and nuts and seeds.

   I personally prefer good-quality butter, olive oil, eggs and occasionally coconut oil or seafood. Strangely, when I received the results from my genome test, it showed that butter and seafood would be the best fat sources for my particular body due to the way I process fats. In addition, my cultural heritage is northern European (Scottish, Irish, English, French) and these were the main fats used in those communities for centuries.

   Many people like coconut oil, but I never seem to feel great after eating it. Then again, as my genetic counsellor said, 'You're not a Pacific Islander!'

3. **Animal protein was eaten daily.** It was obtained predominantly from omega-3-rich fish and seafood, including crustaceans and molluscs, eaten either cooked, raw or fermented; and mammals, birds, reptiles and insects.

   In modern society, we can avail ourselves of ocean fish and seafood, and organic and free-range red meat, chicken and duck. Issues of sustainability should be top of our minds, particularly when it comes to fish consumption. To ensure only sustainable sources of fish are consumed we can download an app to help us make better choices when shopping. We can also select milk, cheese or eggs, preferably from organic, pastured and humanely raised animals. Fermented dairy products such as yoghurt and kefir are also available as a source of probiotics.

Today, increasing numbers of vegans and vegetarians prioritise animal rights among their dietary considerations. Veganism and vegetarianism are very worthy causes, and I personally have immense respect for their commitment to all living creatures. When not followed properly, vegan and vegetarian diets can fail to supply enough complete proteins (essential amino acids), but intake can be upped from foods such as miso, tempeh, amaranth, tofu, lentils, baked beans, linseeds, pumpkin seeds, sesame seeds, nuts and quinoa.

4. **A variety of fruits, land and sea vegetables, nuts and (often sprouted) seeds were consumed.**

In modern society we are limited to only a few varieties of fruits and vegetables relative to the extraordinary numbers of varieties that exist. In addition, many commercially grown versions have lost their flavour as agricultural scientists have sought to increase yields and pest resistance. Seed-saving companies such as Australia's Diggers Club and America's Seed Savers Exchange have made available many different varieties of heritage vegetables and fruits in seed and plant form. People with access to a garden, a few garden pots or a community garden can grow and enjoy these for themselves.

Farmers' markets, organic stores, farm-gate sellers, specialty food stores, Asian supermarkets and online businesses can supply a greater variety of in-season fruits, vegetables, nuts and seeds for consumers who want to venture outside the standard supermarket offering.

5. **Salt was consumed.** People ate salt in necessary amounts, as it was understood to be highly mineralised and essential to health. Salt was obtained from the sea and by following animals to inland salt deposits.

    Today we have access to many different types of mineralised salts from around the world, which we can add to home-cooked meals in pinch-sized amounts. Processed foods contain large amounts of white, processed, demineralised salt as a preservative and to alter taste.

    Being the home blood pressure tracker that I am, I have noticed that when I consume salty processed foods, my blood pressure goes up. Like the great chefs, however, I use unprocessed or mineralised salt in my cooking, and it has no negative effect on my blood pressure.

6. **Nutrient-dense foods were the norm.** These foods contained between two and ten times the essential nutrients of processed foods. Numerous research studies have demonstrated that Westernised populations are low in essential vitamins and minerals due to the poor nutritional content of processed foods.

    Today we are able to access many different types of whole foods and transform them through home cooking, blending or juicing them into nutrient-dense meals capable of delivering high levels of nutrition to our cells. In addition, many cafés and restaurants now provide high-quality nutrient-dense foods.

7. **Plant foods were grown in soil rich in mineral and organic matter.** This enabled the plants to draw in more nutrients, which they transferred to the consuming human or animal.

Today's soils are stripped of nutrients and so farmers often use synthetic fertilisers to feed the plants. Many people are now learning about the art of composting, which is an excellent way to recycle and reduce kitchen waste while creating healthier soils in backyard gardens and in turn more nutrient-dense produce. Composting is also good for the environment, as it reduces landfill.

Books such as *The Complete Idiot's Guide to Composting* by Chris McLaughlin or *The Rodale Book of Composting* are useful guides for anyone wishing to try their hand at developing this skill. There are also websites and YouTube tutorials made by composting enthusiasts who enjoy sharing their knowledge.

Using traditional food preparation, preservation and storage methods

1. **Foods were eaten raw or with minimal cooking.** This meant they retained the maximum amount of nutrition and likely provided bacterial diversity to the microbiome.

   While some people today choose to eat mostly or only raw foods, it's not for everyone. We can, however, choose to include raw foods in our diet by eating lots of fresh salads and some fruit. People interested in testing out raw foods might like to pay a visit to the Plant Gallery, a restaurant in Sydney's Bondi. The owner, a chef, decided to live off a plant-based diet after losing a close friend to cancer. The raw, vegan eatery serves organic, locally sourced food and has plans to grow produce on the premises. All major cities have at least one option in this category, and most other categories you might like to try.

2. **Food was eaten fresh and in season.** People around the world did this until the advent of the ubiquitous supermarket and cold storage.

   Today, most of us can easily access fresh, in-season food from our local supermarkets, green grocers and farmers' markets, or even grow it at home. In-season produce is often more abundant and cheaper than out-of-season produce, and is more likely to be organic and locally grown by smaller local farmers.

3. **Fermented whole foods were included in the diet.** These provided people with plenty of friendly bacteria for their microbiome. Fermented foods help to maintain the microbial balance of the gut, which is the first line of defence in the immune system and responsible for the synthesis of essential nutrients. Fermented foods are a staple in many countries around the world, not just among the indigenous groups studied by Dr Price.

   In today's modern world, fermented foods are both cheap and easy to access. Many recipe books, websites and YouTube videos are available that will teach you how to make ferments in your own home. Fermented foods such as cheese, kefir, sauerkraut, pickles, kimchi, yoghurt, fish, mixed pickled vegetables and kombucha are freely available in specialty food stores and health-food shops. I have even seen kombucha on tap in certain food shops! I personally like to add a teaspoon of apple cider vinegar to my water each day, and to rotate between good-quality yoghurts, kefirs and cheeses.

4. **Food was stored in vessels made from natural materials.** They were made of wood, earthenware, glass or ceramics rather than synthetic materials such as plastics or tins lined with bisphenol A (some of which contain known hormone disruptors).

    While it would seem virtually impossible to avoid all of the plastic, tin and treated paper packaging that houses much of our food supply, we can still use glass, ceramic, earthenware and wooden containers for much of our food storage. It's still possible to buy raw food materials directly from the internet or local suppliers and store the products in natural materials in the home, which cuts down on packaging waste and landfill.

    In addition to the problem of storing foods today is the issue of cooking and bakeware. The Price-Pottenger Nutrition Foundation recommends glass, ceramic, porcelain ware, seasoned cast-iron and stainless steel – no aluminium, silicone or non-stick cookware.

5. **Food was preserved using natural methods.** These techniques, which included drying, salting, pickling, fermenting, freezing (in cold climates) or burying in the soil, were passed down from generation to generation.

    Today we can preserve foods in a very similar fashion by bottling, freezing, sun-drying, air-drying, oven-drying, dehydrating, smoking, canning, freeze-drying and salting – although many of us would probably avoid burying our food in the soil.

Protecting the health of future generations

1. **People consumed the same nutrient-dense whole foods their ancestors had eaten.** The instructions for obtaining, preparing and eating these foods were handed down from generation to generation.

   One of the big differences in today's world is that we have been led to believe that diet 'experts' know what is best for us and so we should simply let them decide what we should eat. This concept is a relatively new one, and it hasn't proven very successful!

   Cultures all across the world received their dietary instructions as part of their cultural inheritance. Elders knew all about which foods were best to eat and how to prepare them for consumption. They knew the medicinal aspects of foods and understood how to use herbs and spices. They knew which plants could harm and which plants were safe. They had knowledge and wisdom that is still unmatched by science.

   It's most unfortunate that many cultures have lost sight of this aspect of their inheritance. Ironically, these cultures now have some of the worst health statistics; they are in desperate need of reclaiming the very wisdom that has been all but lost.

   Today we can look to our own cultural heritage for clues about what worked for our ancestors, and we can also tap into the cultural heritage of other nationalities to experience new flavours, recipes, food preparation and storage techniques.

2. **Special nutrient-dense foods were fed to both men and women of childbearing age.** This helped them prepare for conception, pregnancy, childbirth and lactation, which ensured the best chance for the mother and the baby. Dr Price noted that indigenous populations placed such a high value on providing micronutrients to pregnant women that men would be sent on quests to locate certain plants for use by the mother. Even warring tribes would allow the other to travel into their zone for the purpose of obtaining plants considered essential for conception and pregnancy. In one case described by Dr Price, a group of men would make a dangerous trip down their mountain and into lower lands to obtain a particular plant for use by a single pregnant woman in the tribe.

   Today, many women would be unaware of the importance of preparing their bodies for conception by consuming nutrient-dense, healthy foods and reducing stress well before they become pregnant. Obesity from poor diet affects a woman's ability to conceive and can significantly increase the likelihood of certain birth defects. This indicates a problem that could be fixed by greater education of young women (and men) on the importance of healthy, nutrient-dense food, particularly if they want to create the healthiest children today and into the future.

3. **All infants and young children were breastfed.** This guaranteed the transmission of various microbial components to the baby's immune system, thus assisting the new child to adapt to its unique environment.

Breastfeeding in Western countries has had a chequered history since the increasing medicalisation of childbirth, and the concept of 'scientific motherhood' led doctors to advise women that formula milk was superior to breastmilk. This was despite the fact that breastfeeding was widely understood by public-health workers to be superior. Statistics from the United Kingdom in the early twentieth century noted that the death rate from infant diarrhoea for breastfed babies was 20 per 1000 versus 440 per 1000 for babies fed on cow's milk.

Today, breastfeeding is actively promoted by doctors and public-health workers and the World Health Organization. In Australia, mothers who struggle to breastfeed but don't wish to use formula can receive donated milk from other mothers via the Mothers Milk Bank Charity, an organisation that collects, screens, pasteurises and distributes breastmilk. Milk banks are available in northern New South Wales, south-east and northern Queensland, the ACT, Hobart, Melbourne and Sydney.

4. **Childbirth was spaced by three years at a minimum.** This provided valuable time for the mother to replace her nutritional stores to the highest level possible. This in turn would ensure sufficient nutrition was available for conception and for the growth and protection of the developing baby and later infant. This also enabled optimal milk supply for the infant and for the mother's overall health.

Today, medical science supports the idea of birth spacing: the World Health Organization notes that birth-to-pregnancy intervals of eighteen months or less are linked to greater risk of infant mortality, low birth weight, small size and pre-term delivery. The World Health Organization now recommends a minimum two-year spacing between childbirth and the pursuit of a further pregnancy.

Living a traditional lifestyle

1. **Families and communities ate together.** This gave an opportunity for conversations, laughter, entertainment, problem sharing, information sharing and support, which in turn enhanced the wellbeing of the group.

    Researchers have found that family mealtimes are very beneficial for children in particular, who experience less depression and stress, enjoy better relationships, are less likely to engage in high-risk teenage behaviours, and generally have a better outlook on life. In addition, children who regularly share family meals eat healthier foods with more vegetables and fruits, and less junk food.

    Sharing family mealtimes is less common these days, as today's busy households must adapt to our different work, school and sports schedules. This has rendered the act of eating more of an exercise in refuelling.

    When I was growing up in the 1970s we always ate our evening meals together. In my household today, it's not always possible to eat together due to conflicting schedules, and so we create regular opportunities to eat out and we always share meals on weekends.

2. **Daily exercise was achieved through undertaking daily chores.** These included hunting, gathering foods, working, playing, dancing, and playing sports and games.

   With the exception of hunting (well, for most of us) all of these opportunities for movement and exercise are still available. In addition, we can choose to simply walk the dog, stroll (or stride) around a city or local park, go to a yoga class, join a gym, take up cycling, join a tennis club, do some push-ups against the neighbour's fence or even a high-intensity training session in the back garden.

   The opportunities for exercise are limitless in modern society. The key is to step away from the weapons of mass distraction (computers and other devices, TV and video games), get out into the real world, around real people, and jump straight in to the rhythm of life! No excuses.

3. **Daily sunshine was the norm.** People spent most of their time outdoors, undertaking various activities, and yet skin cancer was evidently not a feature of any of the populations Price visited, including Indigenous Australians (who now do develop skin cancer, although in lower numbers than non-Indigenous Australians).

   In Australia, the experts tell us that two out of three of us will be diagnosed with skin cancer in our lifetime and that we should limit ourselves to a couple of minutes of sun per day, regardless of whether we are vitamin D deficient or not. Vitamin D is converted in the body into calcitriol, a hormone necessary for the expression of 900 genes, many of which are involved the brain. It activates, for example, the enzyme that converts tryptophan to serotonin in the brain. Genes involved in several autoimmune diseases and cancer are also regulated by vitamin D, which is considered to be protective.

Suffice to say, regular sun provides us with natural, free vitamin D, and we should take advantage of it with a commonsense approach that depends on our individual circumstances.

4. **Pure air, water and food were freely available.** Pure air free of pollutants, clean water free of contaminants and chemicals, and clean food grown or pastured in fertile soils and free of chemical fertilisers, farm chemicals, antibiotics, hormones and pharmaceuticals, are very hard to come by in today's world.

Today's consumers are dealing with an increasing number of toxic aspects in their exposome. The natural backlash to this is the 'clean food' and 'clean living' movements, through which people are trying to reclaim an element of purity in their environment and reduce their environmental-toxin load and preserve the environment. They do this by choosing organic, non-GMO, free-range and humanely raised food, drink and personal-care options.

As you can see, there are many ways we can incorporate the various elements of our shared ancestral wisdom back in to our everyday lives and reclaim our health. Dr Weston Price begged us in 1936 to learn of such wisdom and now, 80 years later, for the sake of future generations, the knowledge must be dragged back from the brink before it becomes lost to us forever.

The message was and still is simple.

Mother Nature must be obeyed.

Conclusion

As we have seen, this book started with me being told at a young age that I had a terminal chronic disease that was 'genetic ... just happens to people ... nobody knows how' and being curious enough to discover if that statement was really true. Having learned about the previously chronic-disease-free status of indigenous groups around the world, and the obvious role of sugar, refined wheat and seed oil in destroying their disease resistance and consequently their health, I realised that we as humans were not designed to be weak and disease-riddled – but rather we were being progressively weakened through our diet, and rendered *susceptible to disease*.

While the effect of sugar and refined wheat on the ancient genomes and microbial communities of Price's indigenous research subjects was catastrophic enough, we in the West are now dealing with the effects of exposomes far more damaging and complex than those endured by these people. But the effects are the same, and the sheer scale of the damage being inflicted upon us is truly frightening. Our food supply is dominated by sugar, refined wheat and products filled with omega-6 fats, in addition to other industrial-grade raw materials masquerading as food. For this we can thank the chemical wizardry of the international cadre of 'food scientists', who seek to deceive our tastebuds and in the process are setting us on a path to poor health.

Our dietary guidelines were developed by the agricultural sector, and it would seem that assuring trade in raw materials rather than good science or commitment to creating the healthiest population was and is still at the forefront of dietary decision-making. That the diet experts could get it wrong (and are still getting it wrong) so consistently, and be so unwilling to admit their errors, is astounding. It should not come as a surprise that the failings of the diet experts played quite a significant role in the pharmaceutical sector growing from a US$6 billion dollar sector when the great diet experiment began in 1980 to a US$1 trillion dollar sector just 35 years later.

In addition to the embarrassing litany of failures that can be attributed to the diet experts, we have a globally standardised medical system that limits us to a choice of pharmaceuticals or surgery as a solution to our health problems. This system stems not from a totality of evidence that chemicals and surgery are the best solution for every single health problem every single time, but from a far-reaching decision made by a group of very rich and powerful men 100 years ago. Today, the majority of hospitalisations stem from the effects of the Western diet and our sedentary yet stressful lifestyle. This could not make the mismatch between the actual problem facing medicine and what medicine is limited to offering as a solution any more apparent. Albert Einstein once said that the definition of insanity is doing the same thing over and over again and expecting different results. This could not be truer of the current state of chronic-disease management by the medical system. A bandaid for an epidemic is not going to work.

This particular problem is made infinitely more untenable by the fact that the pharmaceutical, medical and to some degree the health insurance industries are profit-driven and therefore require constant growth, ostensibly to fulfil the shareholder primacy imperative. Constant growth for these industries naturally requires a reliably expanding supply of sick people who are dependent on the products and services marketed by these organisations. This scenario is clearly unsustainable from an economic, workforce planning, social and ethical standpoint. A growth strategy based upon sick people is a strategy doomed to fail. Sick people often have to give up work and hence, instead of generating wealth for the system, become a financial drain that must be offset by the wealth generated by the remaining healthy citizens – who will eventually be few and far between. While this pressure on the system can be absorbed for a short time, it won't last forever – the system will simply collapse under its own weight.

While the mainstream media is busily announcing the latest 'fat gene', 'depression gene' or 'cancer gene', scientists in the field of genetic research have learned that there is a little more to the idea of a disease gene than meets the eye. As it turns out, our genes are designed to code for proteins that build and maintain our bodies – as long as we fuel it with the right stuff. The problem with genes is that they can become faulty and start turning on and off when we would least like them to. One of the key reasons for this is the role of the environment, which means primarily our diet but also our broader exposome. An abundance of scientific research is starting to connect the dots between how our genes react to our nutritional environment, primarily in the field of nutrigenomics and nutrigenetics. This emerging paradigm also lends itself to the concept of nutrient density rather than energy density for better health, which further highlights the gulf between the problem of poor health and medicine's forced reliance on medications and surgery.

In addition to the latest genetic advances are the discoveries relating to our internal microbial communities. This field of research examines everything from the role of our mother's diet, birthing methods, breastfeeding, bacterial diversity and long-term individual diet as likely inputs into whether we develop diseases. Between the role of nutrigenetics and nutrigenomics and the role of our microbial communities in upholding our disease resistance, the idea of maintaining an appropriate personalised diet could not be more important. Researchers are already putting forward the idea that the toilet of the future will be less a hygiene management system and more a urine and faecal analysis unit. It's proposed that the toilet will capture excrement, run a sophisticated analysis on the chemistry and microbial communities contained therein and recommend dietary changes or added nutrition based upon individualised results. It's ironic that quite possibly the 'diet expert' will one day be superseded by a digitally enabled toilet bowl.

In light of the role that sugar, refined wheat and seed oils played in lowering disease resistance among Price's indigenous groups, and their return to health upon reclaiming their indigenous diets, in addition to the modern-day propensity of Western consumers to cut these foods from their diets and report improved health, I decided that these raw materials needed a closer look. Given that I had dramatically improved my own health by removing gluten products and cutting down on sugar, I was interested in finding out what scientists really knew about these foods.

From acting as a key driver of the Trans-Atlantic slave trade to its role in the passing of Britain's anti-slavery laws and its modern-day links to an epidemic of kidney damage – both among the Chichigalpa sugar farmers and its end consumers – sugar's unpalatable history has been anything but dull. While Weston Price's indigenous groups could likely link their terrible dental problems and loss of nutrition to the effects of sugar, the unfolding research into the importance of the microbiome in immunity may be yet another mechanism by which disease susceptibility was induced in these people. In Western populations the news is all bad, starting with the raft of scientific literature pertaining to the role of sugar in inducing metabolic syndrome – a leading forerunner of type 2 diabetes and heart disease, and their numerous unpalatable and yet totally avoidable patient outcomes. Sugar is also being implicated in obesity-linked cancers, many of which went from non-existent to over-represented among Price's indigenous groups.

The gluten-free trend has taken off around the world as people report remission from all kinds of health problems. While the gluten-free brigade is routinely scoffed at by media commentators and diet experts, the rapid growth of the global gluten-free market clearly demonstrates that it's less of a trend and more of a consumer-led change in eating that shows no signs of abating. While coeliac disease is the most obvious of the gluten-related illnesses, the recognition of non-coeliac gluten sensitivity as a distinct entity by the most prominent European and American researchers in the area makes gluten avoidance an acceptable and uncontroversial way to relieve myriad niggling health problems that may fall into this category.

Wheat is also implicated in the obesity and metabolic-syndrome epidemic, and is firmly in the sights of scientists, doctors, patients and investment banks alike. While the diet experts continue with the party line that wholegrains are healthy, even Credit Suisse is rating the low-fat, high-carbohydrate diet a fail with catastrophic consequences for society – a shot across the bow if ever there was one.

In his book *The World Turned Upside Down: The Second Low-carbohydrate Revolution*, biochemist Richard D. Feinman features a 'blog post from a future history of diabetes'. This 'future history' tells the story of a court case brought by a teenage type 2 diabetes patient, Dalton Banting, who was prescribed medications in addition to a diet recommended by the ADA. During court proceedings, it's revealed that on the drug and diet regimen, Banting's symptoms worsened to the point that his foot was amputated. Banting's parents consequently found a new doctor, who prescribed the young Banting a low-carbohydrate diet, which led to rapid and long-term improvement. The parents claimed that Dalton 'should have been offered carbohydrate restriction as an option' for managing his insulin resistance. The final nail in the coffin, which leads to not only a victory for Banting but an avalanche of similar law suits, is a glucometer demonstration in which the ADA diet is shown to produce spikes in blood glucose unlike the low-carbohydrate diet, which shows improved readings.

As the diet experts continue to dismiss low-carbohydrate diets for type 2 diabetes as 'unsustainable' (as opposed to a taxpayer-funded multibillion-dollar healthcare bill and overrun healthcare system, which evidently *is* sustainable), Feinman's 'future history' lawsuit seems more likely with every passing day.

Topping off the whole sorry mess is the omega-6 story. Say no more.

In the course of writing this book I came to learn of the existence of a vast global network of scientific researchers who, unbeknown to me had been hard at work in public- and privately funded laboratories discovering stuff I had never even heard of. The reason I had never heard of these people and their work was simple – I was never meant to. As John Yudkin revealed in his updated edition of *Pure, White and Deadly*, the BNF was designed to stand as a gatekeeper between the average Joe – you and me – and the scientific community. Nutrition science was on a need-to-know basis, and the public simply didn't need to know. From my time wading around in the millions of citations listed in PubMed alone, I realised that nutritional science has moved on – we just weren't told about it. The diet experts and their stakeholders made sure of that.

This top-down, expert-led approach is rapidly passing its use-by date, as the public's trust in our traditional health authorities further erodes with each blatantly industry-friendly, counter-intuitive (in light of our current health crisis) and condescending media release. In their place have risen the micropowers, who have circumvented the fence line and bypassed the traditional authorities before heading straight for the latest scientific literature and reporting their findings to their online communities. Consumers, fed up with diet advice that doesn't stack up and becoming more obese and sick with each passing day, have decided that the micropowers have a better offer and are able to deliver the value they are looking for in a non-judgemental, non-condescending manner. In fact, one of the key features of diet, wellness and health communities is that they enable people to share their struggles in a supportive environment where shaming others, judgement and bullying are simply not tolerated.

The reasons why consumers are seeking new health authorities are clear: they are deeply concerned about the explosion of chronic disease that has happened under the expert advice of the traditional health authorities. The new health authorities appear to be achieving great results, particularly in people who were suffering symptoms of systemic breakdown stemming from a lack of nutrition. Consumers are also increasingly finding themselves dealing with a diagnosis of allergies, food intolerances or autoimmunity (which may have a food or environmental component). For this reason, they are looking outside the box for solutions that meet their needs. This can lead them to find inspiration in community blogs or books, and to purchasing 'free-from' products. People are increasingly aware of the role of the microbiome in maintaining our health and are altering their diets accordingly.

The issue of vested interests providing 'support', financial or otherwise, to the health and diet experts is also worrying. When the director-general of the World Health Organization, Margaret Chan, delivers a one–two punch to the not-so-friendly vested interests that attempt to 'shape the public health policies . . . that affect their products', why should citizens continue to have trust in them? We no longer know who we are dealing with – legitimate scientists, scientists on the industry payroll or big business ensuring that only science of a sympathetic nature is put forward as official 'evidence'. Traditional health authorities cannot seriously expect to continue to enjoy public trust when these links are becoming increasingly apparent.

The obvious nature of our failing physical and mental health on the watch of the traditional health experts has led consumers to seek new ways to adapt to their environment in an effort to become 'antifragile'. This recalibration of the human body and the human spirit has led consumers to turn to wellness social networks, wellness technology, clean and sustainable health solutions, and a renewed emphasis on trust in their interactions and purchasing decisions. These biocitizens are spending big money on looking good and feeling even better, which has led to rapid growth in the wellness industry, particularly the wellness lifestyle businesses led by entrepreneurs aligned with the more mature and evolved 'doing well by doing good' business ethos. People want health solutions, and the creative classes are stepping up to the plate to deliver.

Wellness is still only 'half-invented', and it remains to be seen how the rest of the story will pan out. Might it be possible that the Wayback Machine 2060 will tell a fascinating tale about the time a ragtag bunch of bearded, bike-riding, green-smoothie-chugging hipsters tripped over a group of pioneering, globally dispersed but influential digital Davids and somehow found a way to educate us back from the brink of diet-based destruction towards the prom-ised land of health and wellness? I guess we are in the process of finding out.

Acknowledgements

Firstly, and most importantly, thank you to the unknown person who opted to become an organ donor and in doing so saved my life and gave a little boy back his mother. Without your selfless act, I wouldn't be here and this book would never have been written.

To all the medical professionals who have kept me on this earth and continue to do so – thank you for helping me. I wanted my life and I'm so glad to be here – but my dream is for a world where the terrible toll of preventable chronic disease takes up the least of your valuable time and skills.

A big thank you to my publisher Ingrid Ohlsson who was intrigued enough to give me a chance and valued my manuscript and its message enough to publish it. It is a huge honour.

To Alex Lloyd, my editor who consistently displayed wisdom and insight beyond his years when pulling this book together. Such a great sounding board.

To the broader team at Pan Macmillan who were involved in this book, thank you for your input.

To my agent and friend George Karlov for his endless support through thick and thin, his belief in and commitment to this book never wavered.

To the family and friends who have supported me through the hard slog of writing this book, you know who you are and I will thank you in person.

To Dad, in spite of your own failing health you insisted I not worry and instead focus on finishing this book. Always humble and selfless. Thank you for the life lessons. I miss you – until we meet again.

To all of the courageous writers, bloggers, scientists, food activists, filmmakers, millennium mothers and fathers, health and wellness entrepreneurs, renegade medical professionals, thought leaders, system busters, disrupters, hipsters and anti-fragilistas. Such an inspiration – without our health we, and those who come after us, have nothing and you are lighting the path to a new and better way forward.

Finally, to the fluffy 'Master of the House' who constantly reminded me to step away from the sometimes gut-wrenching business of writing a book of this nature and attend to more important issues, such as chasing birds.

Author's Note

The author would like to thank:

The Price-Pottenger Nutrition Foundation (PPNF) for permission to use and draw upon the work of Dr Weston Price. Readers who would like more information on the travels and work of Dr Price can read his book *Nutrition and Physical Degeneration* or visit the website of PPNF at www.ppnf.org

The American Autoimmune Related Diseases Association (AARDA) for permission to feature their comprehensive list of diseases. Readers who would like more information and descriptions of diseases on this list can visit the AARDA website at www.aarda.org

The World Cancer Research Fund International for permission to feature the diagram pertaining to the influences of food, nutrition, obesity and physical activity on the cancer process, shown in chapter 6.

The 'other' Richard Feinman, Professor of Cell Biology (Biochemistry), State University of New York, for allowing me to use excerpts from his aptly titled book, *The World Turned Upside Down*.

Appendix: Known autoimmune diseases

At the time of writing, this is the current list of autoimmune diseases from by the American Autoimmune Related Diseases Association:

1. Addison's disease
2. Agammaglobulinemia
3. Alopecia areata
4. Amyloidosis
5. Ankylosing spondylitis
6. Anti-GBM/anti-TBM nephritis
7. Antiphospholipid syndrome (APS)
8. Autoimmune hepatitis
9. Autoimmune inner ear disease (AIED)
10. Axonal and neuronal neuropathy (AMAN)
11. Behcet's disease
12. Bullous pemphigoid
13. Castleman disease (CD)
14. Coeliac disease
15. Chagas disease
16. Chronic inflammatory demyelinating polyneuropathy (CIDP)
17. Chronic recurrent multifocal osteomyelitis (CRMO)
18. Churg-Strauss
19. Cicatricial pemphigoid/benign mucosal pemphigoid
20. Cogan's syndrome
21. Cold agglutinin disease

22. Congenital heart block
23. Coxsackie myocarditis
24. CREST disease
25. Crohn's disease
26. Dermatitis herpetiformis
27. Dermatomyositis
28. Devic's disease (neuromyelitis optica)
29. Discoid lupus
30. Dressler's syndrome
31. Endometriosis
32. Eosinophilic oesophagitis
33. Eosinophilic fasciitis
34. Erythema nodosum
35. Essential mixed cryoglobulinemia
36. Evans syndrome
37. Fibromyalgia
38. Fibrosing alveolitis
39. Giant cell arteritis (temporal arteritis)
40. Giant cell myocarditis
41. Glomerulonephritis
42. Goodpasture's syndrome
43. Granulomatosis with polyangiitis (GPA; formerly called Wegener's granulomatosis)
44. Graves' disease
45. Guillain-Barré syndrome
46. Hashimoto's thyroiditis
47. Haemolytic anaemia
48. Henoch-Schonlein purpura (HSP)
49. Herpes gestationis or pemphigoid gestationis (PG)
50. Hypogammaglobulinemia
51. IgA nephropathy
52. IgG4-related sclerosing disease
53. Inclusion body myositis (IBM)
54. Interstitial cystitis (IC)
55. Juvenile arthritis
56. Juvenile diabetes (type 1 diabetes)
57. Juvenile myositis (JM)
58. Kawasaki disease
59. Lambert-Eaton syndrome
60. Leukocytoclastic vasculitis
61. Lichen planus
62. Lichen sclerosus
63. Ligneous conjunctivitis
64. Linear IgA disease (LAD)

65. Lupus (SLE)
66. Lyme disease, chronic
67. Meniere's disease
68. Microscopic polyangiitis (MPA)
69. Mixed connective tissue disease (MCTD)
70. Mooren's ulcer
71. Mucha-Habermann disease
72. Multiple sclerosis (MS)
73. Myasthenia gravis
74. Myositis
75. Narcolepsy
76. Neuromyelitis optica (Devic's)
77. Neutropenia
78. Ocular cicatricial pemphigoid
79. Optic neuritis
80. Palindromic rheumatism (PR)
81. Paediatric autoimmune neuropsychiatric disorders associated with streptococcus (PANDAS)
82. Paraneoplastic cerebellar degeneration (PCD)
83. Paroxysmal nocturnal haemoglobinuria (PNH)
84. Parry–Romberg syndrome
85. Pars planitis (peripheral uveitis)
86. Parsonage–Turner syndrome
87. Pemphigus
88. Peripheral neuropathy
89. Perivenous encephalomyelitis
90. Pernicious anaemia (PA)
91. POEMS syndrome (polyneuropathy, organomegaly, endocrinopathy, monoclonal gammopathy, skin changes)
92. Polyarteritis nodosa
93. Polymyalgia rheumatica
94. Polymyositis
95. Postmyocardial infarction syndrome
96. Postpericardiotomy syndrome
97. Primary biliary cirrhosis
98. Primary sclerosing cholangitis
99. Progesterone dermatitis
100. Psoriasis
101. Psoriatic arthritis
102. Pure red cell aplasia (PRCA)
103. Pyoderma gangrenosum
104. Raynaud's phenomenon
105. Reactive arthritis

106. Reflex sympathetic dystrophy
107. Reiter's syndrome
108. Relapsing polychondritis
109. Restless legs syndrome
110. Retroperitoneal fibrosis
111. Rheumatic fever
112. Rheumatoid arthritis (RA)
113. Sarcoidosis
114. Schmidt syndrome
115. Scleritis
116. Scleroderma
117. Sjögren's syndrome
118. Sperm and testicular autoimmunity
119. Stiff person syndrome (SPS)
120. Subacute bacterial endocarditis (SBE)
121. Susac's syndrome
122. Sympathetic ophthalmia
123. Takayasu's arteritis
124. Temporal arteritis/giant cell arteritis
125. Thrombocytopenic purpura (TTP)
126. Tolosa-Hunt syndrome
127. Transverse myelitis
128. Type 1 diabetes
129. Ulcerative colitis (UC)
130. Undifferentiated connective tissue disease (UCTD)
131. Uveitis
132. Vasculitis
133. Vitiligo
134. Wegener's granulomatosis (granulomatosis with polyangiitis; GPA)

Endnotes

Introduction

12. I was further intrigued when I read . . .: Weston A. Price, *Nutrition and Physical Degeneration*, Price-Pottenger Nutrition Foundation, Lemon Grove, California, 2011 (first published 1939).

13. The loss of immunity to dental caries . . .: ibid., p. 103.

14. Iron, iodine and vitamin A deficiencies . . .: World Health Organization (WHO), 'Getting back to food basics', news release, 12 July 2010, www.wpro.who.int/mediacentre/releases/2010/20100712/en

14. Indigenous Australians are three times . . .: Paul E Norman et al, 'High rates of amputation among indigenous people in Western Australia', *Medical Journal of Australia*, 2012, https://www.mja.com.au/journal/2010/192/7/high-rates-amputation-among-indigenous-people-western-australia

14. Cancer and type 2 diabetes rates . . .: Cancer Monthly, 'Lifestyle changes lead to dramatic cancer increase among Inuit people', 28 October 2008, www.cancermonthly.com/inp/view.asp?ID=228

1 The Wayback Machine

16. 'One can scarcely visualize . . .': Price, *Nutrition and Physical Degeneration*, p. 160.

17. 'In one of the most efficiently organized . . .': ibid., p. 144.

17. 'Dr. Anderson who is in charge . . .': ibid., pp. 119–20.

17. 'An examination of 320 teeth . . .': ibid., p. 133.

18. 'The elderly people were bemoaning . . .': ibid., p. 48.

18. 'My examination of the children . . .': ibid., p. 48.

18. 'The Tahitians are . . . fully conscious . . .': ibid., p. 106.

18. 'Many of the island groups recognize . . . .': ibid., p. 116.

18. 'In their native state they have . . .': ibid., p. 179.

19.	'This group . . . are dependent almost entirely . . .': ibid., pp. 158–59.

19.	'The cook on the government boat . . .': ibid., p. 160.

19.	'On Murray Island . . . the natives . . .': ibid., p. 169.

20.	'He stated that in his thirty-six years . . .': ibid., pp. 83–84.

20.	'The breakdown of these people . . .': ibid., p. 188.

24.	Price notes that the administrators . . .: ibid., p. 432.

24.	Not surprisingly the blood-glucose profile . . .: Tony Kirby, 'Kerin O'Dea: improving the health of indigenous Australians', *The Lancet*, 2012, vol. 380, no. 9846, p. 967.

24.	Researchers have witnessed the same . . .: International Diabetes Federation, '4.7 Western Pacific', *IDF Diabetes Atlas*, 7th edn, IDF, Brussels, 2015, p. 95, www.diabetesatlas.org/resources/2015-atlas.html

25.	The arrival of imported foods . . .: Gary Taubes, *The Diet Delusion*, Vermilion, London, 2008, pp. 136–37.

25.	Access to 'store foods' such as sugar . . .: Staffan Lindeberg, *The Kitava study*, Paleolithic Diet in Medical Nutrition, www.staffanlindeberg.com/TheKitavaStudy. html; Loren Cordain et al., 'Acne vulgaris: a disease of Western civilization', *Archives of Dermatology*, 2002, vol. 138, no. 12, pp. 1584–90, archderm.jamanetwork.com/article.aspx?articleid=479093

26.	Autoimmune disease is breathtakingly rare . . .: Moises Velasquez-Manoff, *An Epidemic of Absence: A New Way of Understanding Allergies and Autoimmune Disease*, Scribner, New York, 2012, p. 10.

26.	Hypertension, at epidemic levels in the West . . .: Michael Gurven et al., 'Does blood pressure inevitably rise with age? Longitudinal evidence among forager-horticulturalists', *Hypertension*, 2012, vol. 60, no. 1, pp. 25–33, hyper.ahajournals.org/content/60/1/25.long

26.	Compare these statistics to Australia . . .: Australian Institute of Health and Welfare, Australian Government, 'A snapshot of rheumatoid arthritis', Bulletin 116, May 2013, http://www.aihw.gov.au/WorkArea/DownloadAsset. aspx?id=60129543377

26.	Lupus is believed to affect over 20,000 . . .: Australian Society of Clinical Immunology and Allergy, 'Systemic Lupus Erythematosus (SLE)', June 2016, http://www.allergy.org.au/images/pcc/ASCIA_PCC_Systemic_Lupus_ Erythematosus_2016.pdf

2 How did *we* get so fat and sick?

29.	According to the World Health Organization . . .: WHO, 'Health topics: noncommunicable diseases', WHO, www.who.int/topics/noncommunicable_diseases/en

29.	People are getting sicker younger . . .: Kate Kelland, 'Chronic disease to cost $47 trillion by 2030: WEF', Reuters, 18 September 2011, www.reuters.com/ article/2011/09/18/us-disease-chronic-costs-idUSTRE78H2IY20110918

30.	According to the World Economic Forum . . .: Henry Taylor, 'Who is the world's biggest employer? The answer might not be what you expect', World Economic Forum, Agenda, 17 June 2015, agenda.weforum.org/2015/06/worlds-10-biggest-employers

30. In early 2014, the World Health Organization . . .: Tim Hume & Jen Christensen, 'WHO: Imminent global cancer "disaster" reflects aging, lifestyle factors', CNN, 5 February 2014, edition.cnn.com/2014/02/04/health/who-world-cancer-report

30. Cancer has now overtaken . . .: Prachi Bhatnagar et al., 'The epidemiology of cardiovascular disease in the UK 2014', *Heart*, 2015, doi:10.1136/ heartjnl-2015-307516, heart.bmj.com/content/early/2015/05/06/ heartjnl-2015-307516.full; Melanie Nichols et al., 'Cardiovascular disease in Europe 2014: epidemiological update', *European Heart Journal*, 2014, vol. 35, no. 42, pp. 2950–59, http://eurheartj.oxfordjournals.org/content/35/42/2950

31. 'Despite exciting advances . . .': WHO International Agency for Research on Cancer, *Global battle against cancer won't be won with treatment alone*, press release no. 224, WHO IARC, Lyon/London, 3 February 2014, www.iarc.fr/en/media-centre/pr/2014/pdfs/pr224_E.pdf

31. The links between obesity . . .: Melina Arnold et al., 'Duration of Adulthood Overweight, Obesity, and Cancer Risk in the Women's Health Initiative: A Longitudinal Study from the United States', *PLOS Medicine*, 16 August 2016, http://journals.plos.org/plosmedicine/article?id=10.1371/journal.pmed.1002081

31. Indeed, one in two British people . . .: 'Lifetime risk of cancer', Cancer Research UK, www.cancerresearchuk.org/health-professional/cancer-statistics/risk/lifetime-risk

32. It shows that we are surrounded . . .: Jess Kirby, 'The causes of cancer you can control', Cancer Research UK, 7 December 2011, scienceblog.cancerresearchuk. org/2011/12/07/the-causes-of-cancer-you-can-control

32. Further research released in 2015 . . .: Song Wu et al., 'Substantial contribution of extrinsic risk factors to cancer development', *Nature*, 2015, vol. 529, no. 7584, pp. 43–47.

33. Chinese consumption of seed oils . . .: 'Obesity and diabetes hit young Chinese', ABC News, 10 February 2015, www.abc.net.au/news/2012–07–24/obesity- diabetes-china/4125964

33. Diabetes costs China around . . .: Darryl Loo, 'China diabetes triples creating $3.2 billion drug market', Bloomberg News, 5 November 2012, www.bloomberg.com/news/articles/2012-11-04/china-diabetes-triples-creating-3- 2-billion-drug-market

34. More rural people . . .: Kounteya Sinha, '44 lakh Indians don't know they are diabetic', *Times of India*, 19 November 2012, timesofindia.indiatimes.com/ india/44-lakh-Indians-dont-know-they-are-diabetic/articleshow/17274366.cms

34. This is because rural Indians . . .: K. Venkaiah et al., 'Diet and nutritional status of rural adolescents in India', *European Journal of Clinical Nutrition*, 2002, vol. 56, no. 11, pp. 1119–25, www.nature.com/ejcn/journal/v56/n11/full/1601457a.html

34. India is also the world's . . .: 'Soybean oil domestic consumption by country in 1000 MT', Index Mundi, 2016, www.indexmundi.com/agriculture/?commodity=soybean- oil&graph=domestic-consumption

35. Soybean oil consumption, which has exploded . . .: Poonamjot Doel et al., 'Soybean oil is more obesogenic and diabetogenic than coconut oil and fructose in mouse:

potential role for liver', *PLOS ONE*, 2015, vol. 10, no. 7, article no. e0132672, journals.plos.org/plosone/article?id=10.1371/journal.pone.0132672

35.   In addition, researchers have discovered . . .: 'Type 3 diabetes', Diabetes.co.uk, www.diabetes.co.uk/type3-diabetes.html

35.   In 2015 American researchers . . .: 'New link between diabetes, Alzheimer's found', Science Daily, 4 May 2015, www.sciencedaily.com/releases/2016/06/160621112107. htm; 'High blood sugar makes Alzheimer's plaque more toxic to the brain', Science Daily, 29 October 2013, www.sciencedaily.com/releases/2013/10/131029090345.htm

36.   More than 400 trials . . .: Jeffrey L. Cummings et al., 'Alzheimer's disease drug-development pipeline: few candidates, frequent failures', *Alzheimer's Research and Therapy*, 2014, vol. 6, article no. 37, alzres.biomedcentral.com/articles/10.1186/alzrt269

36.   The outlook for females . . .: 'One in three people born in 2015 will develop dementia, new analysis shows', Alzheimer's Research UK, 21 September 2015, www.alzheimersresearchuk.org/one-in-three-2015-develop-dementia

38.   It's believed the real figure . . .: American Autoimmune Related Diseases Association & National Coalition of Autoimmune Patient Groups, *The Cost Burden of Autoimmune Disease: The Latest Front in the War on Healthcare Spending*, AARDA, Eastpointe, Michigan, 2011, p. 3, www.diabetesed.net/page/_files/autoimmune-diseases.pdf

38.   In addition, the NIH estimates . . .: 'Autoimmune statistics', AARDA, www.aarda.org/autoimmune-information/autoimmune-statistics

38.   In Finalnd the incidence of type 1 . . .: AARDA & NCAPG, *The Cost Burden of Autoimmune Disease*, p. 4.

38.   Reality TV star Kim Kardashian . . .: Crystal Bell, 'Kim Kardashian diagnosed with psoriasis', Huffington Post, 25 July 2011, www.huffingtonpost.com/2011/07/25/kim-kardashian-diagnosed-_n_908412.html; Leezel Tanglao, 'Venus Williams withdraws from US Open due to Sjogren's syndrome', ABC News (US), 1 September 2011, abcnews.go.com/blogs/health/2011/08/31/venus-williams-withdraws-from-u-s-open-due-to-sjogrens-syndrome

38.   In 2015, pop singer Selena Gomez . . .: Stephanie Castillo, 'Selena Gomez reveals rare disease: what is lupus, and will chemotherapy work for you, too?', Medical Daily, 11 October 2015, www.medicaldaily.com/selena-gomez-reveals-rare-disease-what-lupus-and-will-chemotherapy-work-you-too-356776

38.   Scientists have found that autoimmune . . .: Amy D. Proal et al., 'Inflammatory Disease and the human microbiome', *Discovery Medicine*, 2014, vol. 17, no. 95, pp. 257–65, www.discoverymedicine.com/Amy-D-Proal/2014/05/22/inflammatory-disease-and-the-human-microbiome

38.   It's thus worth noting . . .: Troy Brown, '100 best-selling, most prescribed branded drugs through March', Medscape, 6 May 2015, www.medscape.com/viewarticle/844317

39.   Autoimmune diseases have a genetic precursor . . .: AARDA, *New Trends in Autoimmunity for Patients, Researchers and the American Public: Highlights from 'The State of Autoimmune Disease: A National Summit'*, AARDA, Eastpointe, Michigan, 2015, www.aarda.org/wp-content/uploads/2015/12/HighlightsFromSummitMarch20151.pdf

41. While the exact genetic and environmental . . .: Kenneth M. Pollard, 'Environment, autoantibodies, and autoimmunity', *Frontiers in Immunology*, 2015, vol. 6, article no. 60, www.ncbi.nlm.nih.gov/pmc/articles/PMC4324151; Noel R. Rose, 'Autoimmunity: the common thread', AARDA, www.aarda.org/wp-content/uploads/2013/09/common_thread_textalign.indd_.pdf

41. This is interesting . . .: Esther Han, 'Nanotechnology found in popular foods, despite repeated denials by regulator', *The Age*, 17 September 2015, www.theage.com.au/business/retail/nanotechnology-found-in-popular-foods-despite-repeated-denials-by-regulator-20150916-gjnqgj.html; Robert Reed et al., 'Detecting engineered nanomaterials in processed foods from Australia: final report', Friends of the Earth Emerging Tech Project, 18 August 2015, p. 2, emergingtech.foe.org.au/wp-content/uploads/2015/09/FoE-Aus-Report-Final-web.pdf

41. FOE has since called . . .: 'Study raises more questions about the use of nanoparticles in food', Friends of the Earth Emerging Tech Project, 25 September 2015, emergingtech.foe.org.au/new-study-raises-further-questions-about-the-safety-of-nanoparticles-in-food

41. Given the world's bestselling herbicide . . .: WHO IARC, 'IARC Monographs Volume 112: evaluation of five organophosphate insecticides and herbicides', WHO IARC, 20 March 2015, www.iarc.fr/en/media-centre/iarcnews/pdf/MonographVolume112.pdf

42. Glyphosate acts as an antibiotic . . .: John P. Myers et al., 'Concerns over use of glyphosate-based herbicides and risks associated with exposures: a consensus statement', *Environmental Health*, 2016, vol. 15, article no. 19, ehjournal.biomedcentral.com/articles/10.1186/s12940-016-0117-0

42. More than 60 per cent of breads . . .: Damian Carrington, 'Over 60% of breads sold in the UK contain pesticide residues, tests show', *The Guardian*, 17 July 2014, www.theguardian.com/environment/2014/jul/17/pesticide-residue-breads-uk-crops; 'Pesticide linked to cancer found in top German beers', The Local, 25 February 2016, www.thelocal.de/20160225/tests-find-cancer-inducing-chemical-in-german-beers; Myers et al., 'Concerns over use of glyphosate-based herbicides and risks associated with exposures'.

43. CFS, also known as . . .: University of Bristol, '1 in 50 16-year-olds affected by chronic fatigue syndrome', press release, 25 January 2016, www.bristol.ac.uk/alspac/news/2016/chronic-fatigue-syndrome.html

44. Known as the 'ABCDs' . . .: Sophia Murphy et al., *Cereal Secrets: The World's Largest Grain Traders and Global Agriculture*, Oxfam Research Reports, Oxford, 2012, p. 9, www.oxfam.org/sites/www.oxfam.org/files/file_attachments/rr-cereal-secrets-grain-traders-agriculture-30082012-en_4.pdf

45. Brazil produces nearly half . . .: Sarah McFarlane & Reese Ewing, 'Update 2-Cargill, Copersucar to form world's largest no. 1 sugar trader', Reuters, 27 March 2014, www.reuters.com/article/2014/03/27/cargill-sugar-idUSL5N0MO3O220140327

46. Not content to control . . .: Murphy et al., *Cereal Secrets*, p. 5.

46.   These companies are also rarely . . .: Murphy et al., *Cereal Secrets*, p. 5; Oxfam, 'Behind the brands: food justice and the 'big 10' food and beverage companies', Oxfam Briefing Paper no. 166, 26 February 2013, p. 2, www.oxfam.org/sites/www. oxfam.org/files/bp166-behind-the-brands-260213-en.pdf

47.   Moss details the extraordinarily . . .: Michael Moss, *Salt, Sugar, Fat: How the Food Giants Hooked Us*, Random House, New York, 2013.

47.   This magical combination . . .: Oxfam, 'Behind the brands', p. 6.

47.   According to Moss, at a meeting . . .: Moss, *Salt, Sugar, Fat*, pp. 7–8.

49.   Sales of carbonated drinks . . .: Amy Guthrie, 'Survey shows Mexicans drinking less soda after tax', *Wall Street Journal*, 13 October 2014, www.wsj.com/articles/ survey-shows-mexicans-drinking-less-soda-after-tax-1413226009

49.   Lack of access to clean drinking water . . .: Guthrie, 'Survey shows Mexicans drinking less soda after tax'.

49.   In November 2014 Berkeley . . .: Victoria Guerra, 'Sugar tax UK: Life Science Minister suggests unhealthy sugary foods COULD face taxes', Food World News, 23 May 2015, www.foodworldnews.com/articles/19123/20150523/sugar-tax-uk- life-science-minister-suggests-unhealthy-sugary-foods-could-face-taxes.htm

50.   In the United Kingdom, where . . .: Guerra, 'Sugar tax UK'.

50.   Freeman's assertion was quickly rebuffed . . .: Press Association, 'Government rules out "sugar tax"', *Daily Mail* (Australia), 23 May 2015, www.dailymail.co.uk/wires/ pa/article-3092152/Tax-unhealthy-food-cut-obesity.html

51.   Interestingly, David Cameron, like Jeb Bush . . .: Shaun Smillie, 'How Tim Noakes has caused a drop in sales of rice, pasta and bread', *Rand Daily Mail*, 11 June 2015, www.rdm.co.za/lifestyle/2015/06/10/how-tim-noakes-has-caused-a-drop-in- sales-of-rice-pasta-and-bread

52.   Evidently, many parents were in denial . . .: Jack Doyle, 'More than 70 morbidly obese children taken into care due to concerns over their health', *Daily Mail* (Australia), 28 February 2014, www.dailymail.co.uk/news/article-2569922/More- 70-morbidly-obese-children-overfed-parents-taken-care.html

52.   A RAND Corporation report . . .: Richard A. Rettig et al., *Chronic Kidney Disease: A Quiet Revolution in Nephrology: Six Case Studies*, 2010, Rand Corporation, Santa Monica, California, p. 69, www.rand.org/pubs/technical_ reports/TR826.html

53.   With a background in public health . . .: Luise Light, *What to Eat: The Ten Things You Really Need to Know to Eat Well and Be Healthy*, McGraw-Hill, New York, 2006, p. 13.

55.   Light's predictions eventually . . .: 'Adult obesity in the United States', The State of Obesity, 15 September 2015, stateofobesity.org/adult-obesity

56.   Science writer and British Conservative peer . . .: Chris Brooke, 'Why butter and eggs won't kill us after all: flawed science triggers U-turn on cholesterol fears', *Daily Mail* (Australia), 26 May 2015, http://www.dailymail.co.uk/health/ article-3096634/Why-butter-eggs-won-t-kill-Flawed-science-triggers-U-turn- cholesterol-fears.html

56. In September 2015 the research arm . . .: Stefano Natella et al., *Fat: The New Health Paradigm*, Credit Suisse Research Institute, Zurich, 2015, p. 20, https://www.credit-suisse.com/au/en/about-us/research/research-institute/publications.html

57. Credit Suisse noted that . . .: Natella, *Fat*, p. 6.

58. In addition, the 2015 Dietary Guidelines . . .: 'Stop the National Academy of Medicine from stacking the panel on dietary guidelines with government insiders', Nutrition Coalition, http://www.nutrition-coalition.org/stop-the-national-academy-of-medicine-from-stacking-the-panel-on-dietary-guidelines-with-government-insiders/

58. In recognition of the fact . . .: 'Mayo clinic healthy weight pyramid', Mayo Clinic, www.mayoclinic.org/healthy-lifestyle/weight-loss/in-depth/weight-loss/itt-20084941

58. The not-for-profit organisation Oldways . . .: 'Traditional diets', Oldways, oldwayspt.org/traditional-diets

59. Sadly, we have allowed . . .: Bonnie Malkin, 'Australian teenagers facing lower life expectancy than their parents', *The Telegraph* (London), 9 February 2011, www.telegraph.co.uk/news/worldnews/australiaandthepacific/australia/8313217/Australian-teenagers-facing-lower-life-expectancy-than-their-parents.html

3 The industry of sickness

61. But not even John D. Rockefeller . . .: Y. Claire Wang et al., 'Health and economic burden of the projected obesity trends in the USA and the UK', *The Lancet*, 2011, vol. 378, no. 9793, pp. 815–25.

62. Boldly referring to their own techniques . . .: E. Richard Brown, *Rockefeller Medicine Men: Medicine and Capitalism in America*, University of California Press, Berkeley, p. 62.

62. Increasingly fearful of the tendency . . .: Brown, *Rockefeller Medicine Men*, p. 62.

63. He was also the subject of . . .: Paulo Lionni, *The Leipzig Connection*, Heron Books, Sheridan, Oregon, 1993, p. 44.

63. An arrangement was created . . .: Ibid., p. 50.

64. In 1910, the Carnegie Foundation . . .: Abraham Flexner, *Medical Education in the United States and Canada*, Carnegie Foundation for the Advancement of Teaching, New York, 1910.

64. Gates offered to make a donation . . .: Lionni, *The Leipzig Connection*, p. 70.

64. Flexner left the Carnegie Foundation . . .: Ibid., p. 71.

65. In the allocation of these funds . . .: Brown, *Rockefeller Medicine Men*, p. 11.

65. Sympathetic media connections . . .: Thomas P. Duffy, 'The Flexner Report – 100 years later', *Yale Journal of Biology and Medicine*, 2011, vol. 84, no. 3, pp. 269–76.

65. The General Education Board also allocated . . .: Brown, *Rockefeller Medicine Men*, p. 49.

65. Gates genuinely believed . . .: Brown, *Rockefeller Medicine Men*, p. 129.

65. The industry reforms, which were by no means . . .: Duffy, 'The Flexner Report – 100 years later'.

66.   Today, the global revenue generated . . .: 'Revenue of the worldwide pharmaceutical market from 2001 to 2014 (in billion U.S. dollars)', Statista, 2016, www.statista.com/statistics/263102/pharmaceutical-market-worldwide-revenue-since-2001

67.   In 1970, the *New York Times Magazine* . . .: Milton Friedman, 'The social responsibility of business is to increase its profits', *New York Times Magazine*, 13 September 1970, www.colorado.edu/studentgroups/libertarians/issues/friedman-soc-resp-business.html

67.   'A corporate executive is an employee . . .': Ibid.

68.   'to use its resources and engage in activities . . .': Ibid.

69.   In addition, the idea of placing shareholders . . .: Lynn A. Stout, 'The problem of corporate purpose', *Issues in Governance Studies*, no. 48, June 2012, p. 1, https://www.brookings.edu/wp-content/uploads/2016/06/Stout_Corporate-Issues.pdf

69.   'There is no legal duty to maximise . . .': Lynn Stout, interviewed by Justin O'Brien, 'Corporate governance – what do shareholders really value?', University of New South Wales TV, 4 December 2011, www.youtube.com/watch?v=X2t2bES5y9s

69.   In addition, a focus on shareholders . . .: Lynn Stout, *The Shareholder Value Myth: How Putting Shareholders First Harms Investors, Corporations, and the Public*, Berrett-Koehler Publishers, San Francisco, 2012, p. vi.

70.   Shkreli described the price hike . . .: Michael E. Miller, '"Pharma bro" Martin Shkreli arrested by the FBI on security fraud charges', *The Age*, 18 December 2015, www.theage.com.au/business/world-business/pharma-bro-martin-shkreli-arrested-by-the-fbi-on-security-fraud-charges-20151217-glqf3u.html

71.   'it is likely that the interests . . .': Leo E. Strine Jnr, 'Can we do better by ordinary investors? A pragmatic reaction to the dueling ideological mythologists of corporate law', *Columbia Law Review*, 2014, vol. 114, no. 2, pp. 449, 450–502, columbialawreview.org/wp-content/uploads/2016/04/Strine-L..pdf

71.   'When the pressure to deliver profits . . .': Leo E. Strine Jnr, 'Our continuing struggle with the idea that for-profit corporations seek profit', *Wake Forest Law Review*, 2012, vol. 47, pp. 135–72, wakeforestlawreview.com/wp-content/uploads/2014/10/Strine_LawReview_4.12.pdf

73.   While the US National Academy of Sciences . . .: Kelly M. Adams et al., 'Nutrition education in U.S. medical schools: latest update of a national survey', *Academic Medicine*, 2010, vol. 85, no. 9, pp. 1537–42, journals.lww.com/academicmedicine/Fulltext/2010/09000/Nutrition_Education_in_U_S__Medical_Schools_.30.aspx

73.   'Appropriate public education . . .': US Senate Select Committee on Nutrition and Human Needs, 'Dietary goals for the United States', 95th Congress, 1st Session, February 1977, zerodisease.com/archive/Dietary_Goals_For_The_United_States.pdf

74.   Geiger is famously reputed to have replied . . .: B.J. Healy & R.S. Zimmerman, *The New World of Health Promotion: New Program Development, Implementation and Evaluation*, Jones and Bartlett Publishers, Massachusetts, 2010, p.164.

75.   Professor Yehuda Shoenfeld, head . . .: Yehuda Shoenfeld et al., 'The autoimmunologist: geoepidemiology, a new centre of gravity and a prime time for autoimmunity', *Journal of Autoimmunity*, vol. 31, no. 4, 2008, pp. 325–30.

76. For example GMHBA offers . . .: 'Your health', GMHBA, www.gmhba.com.au/health-community/health-programs; 'Living well programs', BUPA, www.bupa.com.au/health-and-wellness/programs-and-support/living-well-programs/living-well-programs

78. In 2014, the Aspen Institute's . . .: Aspen Institute Business and Society Program, 'Unpacking corporate purpose: a report on the beliefs of executives, investors and scholars', May 2014, assets.aspeninstitute.org/content/uploads/files/content/upload/Unpacking_Corporate_Purpose_May_2014_0.pdf

80. Strine suggests that getting this model right . . .: Leo E. Strine Jnr, 'Making it easier for directors to "do the right thing"?', *Harvard Business Law Review*, 2014, vol. 4, no. 2, p. 235–53, www.hblr.org/wp-content/uploads/2014/10/4.2-5.-Strine-Do-the-Right-Thing.pdf

4 Not everything is genetic

83. In later years he wrote extensively . . .: James G. Hirsch & Carol L. Moberg, 'René Jules Dubois: February 20, 1901–February 20, 1982', *Biographical Memoirs*, 1989, vol. 58, pp. 147–48

83. His detailed knowledge of pathogens . . .: Hirsch & Moberg, 'René Jules Dubos', p. 141.

84. Dubos's research gave him unique . . .: Brown, *Rockefeller Medicine Men*, p. 235.

84. Decades ahead of his time . . .: Hirsch & Moberg, 'René Jules Dubos', p. 145

84. In recent years, it has been confirmed . . .: Isabel Moreno-Indias et al., 'Impact of the gut microbiota on the development of obesity and type 2 diabetes mellitus', *Frontiers in Microbiology*, 2014, vol. 5, article no. 190.

84. Indeed, environmental factors . . .: Moreno-Indias et al., 'Impact of the gut microbiota on the development of obesity and type 2 diabetes mellitus'.

84. In his professional life, René Dubos . . .: Hirsch & Moberg, 'René Jules Dubos', p. 141.

84. Dubos also published many books . . .: Ibid., p. 145.

85. Unfortunately, many sick or unhealthy people . . .: Jeremy A. Kaplan, 'Researchers find the "liberal gene"', Fox News, 28 October 2010, www.foxnews.com/scitech/2010/10/28/researchers-liberal-gene-genetics-politics

85. Despite studying the genes of thousands . . .: Teri A. Manolio et al., 'Finding the missing heritability of complex diseases', *Nature*, 2009, vol. 461, no. 7265, pp. 747–53.

86. In 1944, Avery, McCarty and McLeod . . .: Robert Cook-Deegan, *The Gene Wars: Science, Politics, and the Human Genome*, W.W. Norton and Co., New York, 1995, p. 10.

87. Watson and Crick published their paper . . .: James D. Watson & Francis H.C. Crick, 'Molecular structure of nucleic acids: a structure for deoxyribose nucleic acid', *Nature*, 1953, vol. 171, no. 4356, www.nature.com/nature/dna50/watsoncrick.pdf

88. By 2001, Dr Francis Collins . . .: 'An overview of the Human Genome Project', National Human Genome Research Institute, 11 May 2016, www.genome.gov/12011238/an-overview-of-the-human-genome-project

88. None of these is more perplexing . . .: Manolio et al., 'Finding the missing heritability of complex diseases'.

89. The Human Genome Project estimated . . .: 'The mouse genome and the measure of man', NIH News Advisory, National Human Genome Research Institute, December 2002, www.genome.gov/10005831/2002-release-the-mouse-genome-and-the-measure-of-man

92. Collectin proteins feature a lectin . . .: 'COLEC gene family', Genetics Home Reference, US National Library of Medicine, http://www.genenames.org/cgi-bin/genefamilies/set/491

92. One of the COLEC gene family . . .: Q. Ashton Acton (ed.), *Membrane Proteins: Advances in Research and Application*, Scholarly Editions, Atlanta, Georgia, 2013, p. 166.

93. MBL deficiency has been reported . . .: Ibid., p. 166.

93. This makes these people very susceptible . . .: Ian C. Michelow et al., 'High-dose mannose-binding lectin therapy for Ebola virus infection', *Journal of Infectious Diseases*, 2011, vol. 203, no. 2, pp. 175–79.

93. MBL deficiency is associated with . . .: Beili Shi et al., 'Identification of mannose-binding lectin as a mechanism in progressive immunoglobulin A nephropathy', *International Journal of Experimental Pathology*, 2015, vol. 8, no. 2, pp. 1889–99, www.ncbi.nlm.nih.gov/pmc/articles/PMC4396276

94. Variations such as MBL2 . . .: 'What are single nucleotide polymorphisms (SNPs)?', Genetics Home Reference, US National Library of Medicine, 19 July 2016, ghr.nlm.nih.gov/handbook/genomicresearch/snp; 'Glossary'; SNPedia, 10 June 2016, snpedia.com/index.php/Glossary

94. Appropriate methylation is critical . . .: John Milner et al., 'Nutrigenomics', in Maxine Weinstein et al. (eds), *Biosocial Surveys*, National Academies Press, Washington, DC, 2008, pp. 278–303, www.nap.edu/read/11939/chapter/19

94. These epigenetic markers . . .: 'What are single nucleotide polymorphisms (SNPs)?'.

95. This means perhaps that relying on genetics . . .: Evan E. Eichler et al., 'Missing heritability and strategies for finding the underlying causes of complex disease', *Nature Reviews Genetics*, 2010, vol. 11, no. 6, pp. 446–50.

95. The 'exposome' has been proposed . . .: Martine Vrijheid, 'The exposome: a new paradigm to study the impact of the environment on health', *Thorax*, 2014, vol. 69, no. 9, pp. 876–78.

96. Nutrigenetics refers to the role . . .: Claude Bouchard & Jose M. Ordovas, '*Recent Advances in Nutrigenetics and Nutrigenomics*, Academic Press, London, 2012, p. 2.

96. Specifically, nutrigenetics looks at . . .: Michael Fenech et al., 'Nutrigenetics and nutrigenomics: viewpoints on the current status and applications in nutrition research and practice', *Journal Nutrigenetics and Nutrigenomics*, 2011, vol. 4, no. 2, pp. 69–89.

96. For example, abnormal DNA . . .: Henry Osiecki, *The Nutrient Bible*, 9th edn, Bio Concepts Publishing, Brisbane, 2014, p. 416.

96. Nutrigenomics refers to the effect . . .: Bouchard & Ordovas, *Recent Advances in Nutrigenetics and Nutrigenomics*, p. 2.

96. This includes genome instability . . .: Fenech et al., 'Nutrigenetics and nutrigenomics'.

97. In addition, individual differences may exist . . .: Claude Bouchard & Jose M. Ordovas, 'Fundamentals of nutrigenetics and nutrigenomics', *Progress in Molecular Biology and Translational Science*, 2012, vol. 108, pp. 1–15.

97. Only 2 per cent of Europeans . . .: Carl Zimmer, 'Inuit study adds twist to omega-3 fatty acid's health story', *New York Times*, 17 September 2015, www.nytimes. com/2015/09/22/science/inuit-study-adds-twist-to-omega-3-fatty-acids-health-story. html?_r=0

97. Nutrition may impact health directly . . .: Fenech et al., 'Nutrigenetics and nutrigenomics'.

97. The health benefits associated with nutrients . . .: Ibid.

97. Dietary intervention based upon . . .: Jim Kaput & Raymond L. Rodriguez, 'Nutritional genomics: the next frontier in the postgenomic era', *Physiological Genomics*, 2004, vol. 16, no. 2, pp. 166–77, physiolgenomics.physiology.org/ content/16/2/166

98. The condition is screened for . . .: Kaput & Rodriguez, 'Nutritional genomics', p. 168.

98. The condition is managed . . .: F.D. Martinez, 'Genes, environments, development and asthma: a reappraisal', *European Respiratory Journal*, 2007, vol. 29, no. 1, pp. 179–84, erj.ersjournals.com/content/29/1/179

100. An analysis of Swiss children . . .: Barbara Troesch et al., 'Increased intake of foods with high nutrient density can help to break the intergenerational cycle of malnutrition and obesity', *Nutrients*, 2015, vol. 7, no. 7, pp. 6016–37, www.mdpi. com/2072-6643/7/7/5266/htm

101. The group concluded that a shift . . .: Ibid., p. 6025.

101. In a 2015 review paper titled 'What if . . .: Julia J. Rucklidge et al., 'What if nutrients could treat mental illness?', *Australian and New Zealand Journal of Psychiatry*, 2015, vol. 49, no. 5, pp. 407–408, anp.sagepub.com/content/49/5/407.full

101. This reflects other research . . .: Ibid.

102. A 2015 systematic review . . .: Andrea Amerio et al., 'Carcinogenicity of psychotropic drugs: a systematic review of US Food and Drug Administration–required preclinical in vivo studies', *Australian and New Zealand Journal of Psychiatry*, 2015, vol. 49, no. 8, pp. 686–96, anp.sagepub.com/content/49/8/686.long

104. Not only did the first bowel movement . . .: Scott F. Gilbert, 'A holobiont birth narrative: the epigenetic transmission of the human microbiome', *Frontiers in Genetics*, 2014, vol. 5, article no. 282, www.ncbi.nlm.nih.gov/pmc/articles/ PMC4137224

105. No such transmission was observed . . .: Linda V. Thomas et al., 'Exploring the influence of the gut microbiota and probiotics on health: a symposium report', *British Journal of Nutrition*, 2014, vol. 112, supplement S1, pp. S1– S18, journals.cambridge.org/action/displayAbstract?fromPage=online&aid =9288445&fulltextType=RA&fileId=S0007114514001275

105. They provide essential vitamins . . .: Gilbert, 'A holobiont birth narrative'.

105. This essential colonisation of the newborn . . .: Ibid.

105. In one study of Iranian babies . . .: Mansoureh Taghizadeh et al., 'The influence
      of impact delivery mode, lactation time, infant gender, maternal age and rural
      or urban life on total number of *Lactobacillus* in breast milk Isfahan – Iran',
      Advanced Biomedical Research, 2015, vol. 4, article no. 141, www.advbiores.net/
      article.asp?issn=2277-9175;year=2015;volume=4;issue=1;spage=141;epage=141;aul
      ast=Taghizadeh

105. Researchers already know that caesarean babies . . .: Peris M. Munyaka et al.,
      'External influence of early childhood establishment of gut microbiota and
      subsequent health implications', *Frontiers in Pediatrics*, 2014, vol. 2, article no.
      109, journal.frontiersin.org/article/10.3389/fped.2014.00109/full; Noah Voreades
      et al., 'Diet and the development of the human intestinal microbiome', *Frontiers in
      Microbiology*, 2014, vol. 5, article no. 494, journal.frontiersin.org/article/10.3389/
      fmicb.2014.00494/full

106. Given that the gut is a primary . . .: Vijay C. Antharam et al., 'Intestinal dysbiosis
      and depletion of butyrogenic bacteria in *Clostridium difficile* infection and
      nosocomial diarrhea', *Journal of Clinical Microbiology*, 2013, vol. 51, no. 9,
      pp. 2884–92, jcm.asm.org/content/51/9/2884.long

106. In addition, the sugars in breastmilk . . .: Gilbert, 'A holobiont birth narrative'.

106. Breastmilk itself has been found . . .: Katherine M. Hunt et al., 'Characterisation
      of the diversity and temporal stability of bacterial communities in human
      milk', *PLoS ONE*, vol. 6, no. 6, article no. e21313, journals.plos.org/plosone/
      article?id=10.1371/journal.pone.0021313

106. None of these are present . . .: Zhenjiang Xu & Rob Knight, 'Dietary effects
      of human microbiome diversity', *British Journal of Nutrition*, 2015, vol. 113,
      supplement, pp. S1–S5, www.ncbi.nlm.nih.gov/pmc/articles/PMC4405705

106. Research from Iran has shown . . .: Taghizadeh et al., 'The influence of impact
      delivery mode, lactation time, infant gender, maternal age and rural or urban life on
      total number of *Lactobacillus* in breast milk Isfahan – Iran'.

106. The Yakult researchers noted that . . .: Thomas et al., 'Exploring the influence of the
      gut microbiota and probiotics on health'.

106. While vaginally delivered babies . . .: Maria G. Dominguez-Bello et al.,
      'Delivery mode shapes the acquisition and structure of the initial microbiota
      across multiple body habitats in newborns', *Proceeds of the National
      Academy of Sciences*, 2010, vol. 107, no. 26, pp. 11971–75, www.pnas.org/
      content/107/26/11971.long

107. Early results demonstrated that regardless . . .: Thomas et al., 'Exploring the
      influence of the gut microbiota and probiotics on health'.

107. In addition, a study into the gut microbiome . . .: Amanda R. Highet et al., 'Gut
      microbiome in sudden infant death syndrome (SIDS) differs from that in healthy
      comparison babies and offers an explanation for the risk factor of prone position',
      International Journal Medical Microbiology, 2014, vol. 304, no. 5, pp. 735–41.

107. Research has suggested that long-term . . .: Xu & Knight, 'Dietary effects of human
      microbiome diversity'.

107. The Bacteroidetes and Firmicutes . . .: D. Mariat et al., 'The Firmicutes/
Bacteroidetes ratio of the human microbiota changes with age', *BMC
Microbiology*, 2009, vol. 9, article no. 123, bmcmicrobiol.biomedcentral.com/
articles/10.1186/1471-2180-9-123

108. Faecal analysis of the microbiota . . .: Arancha Hevia et al., 'Intestinal dysbiosis
associated with systemic lupus erythematosus', *mBio*, 2014, vol. 5, no. 5,
article no. e01548-14, www.ncbi.nlm.nih.gov/pmc/articles/PMC4196225/pdf/
mBio.01548–14.pdf

108. Bacteroidetes are a very diverse group . . .: François Thomas et al., 'Environmental
and gut Bacteroidetes: the food connection', *Frontiers in Microbiology*, 2011,
vol. 2, no. 93, journal.frontiersin.org/article/10.3389/fmicb.2011.00093/full

108. Butyrate itself is understood . . .: Roberto B. Canani et al., 'Potential beneficial
effects of butyrate in intestinal and extraintestinal diseases', *World Journal of
Gastroenterology*, 2011, vol. 17, no. 12, pp. 1519–28, www.wjgnet.com/1007-
9327/full/v17/i12/1519.htm

108. Firmicutes, also known as . . .: Farhana Shamin et al., 'Firmicutes dominate the
bacterial taxa within sugar-cane processing plants', *Scientific Reports*, 2013, vol. 3,
article no. 3107, www.nature.com/articles/srep03107

110. Even more fascinating is that . . .: Jose C. Clemente et al., 'The microbiome of
uncontacted Amerindians', *Science Advances*, 2015, vol. 1, article no. 3, advances.
sciencemag.org/content/1/3/e1500183.full

110. This skin microbiota was in stark . . .: Ibid.

110. Fewer species means a lower number . . .: Thomas et al., 'Exploring the influence of
the gut microbiota and probiotics on health'.

111. Diseases associated with low species . . .: Ibid.

117. Zinc deficiency is considered . . .: Jerome Nriagu, 'Zinc deficiency in human health',
Elsevier, Amsterdam, 2007, http://www.extranet.elsevier.com/homepage_about/
mrwd/nvrn/Zinc%20Deficiency%20in%20Humans.pdf

117. Common foods such as wheat . . .: Osiecki, *The Nutrient Bible*, p. 213.

117. In addition, adequate vitamin C levels . . .: Hua Zhong et al., 'Overexpression
of hypoxia-inducible factor 1α in common human cancers and their metastases',
Cancer Research, 1999, vol. 59, no. 22, pp. 5830–35, cancerres.aacrjournals.
org/content/59/22/5830.long; Caroline Kuiper et al., 'Low ascorbate levels are
associated with increased hypoxia-inducible factor-1 activity and an aggressive
tumor phenotype in endometrial cancer', *Cancer Research*, 2010, vol. 70, no. 14,
pp. 5749–58, cancerres.aacrjournals.org/content/70/14/5749.long

5 Can seed oils make us sick?

124. Linoleic acid occurs in high quantities . . .: Mary G. Enig, *Know Your Fats: The
Complete Primer for Understanding the Nutrition of Fats, Oils and Cholesterol*,
2000, Bethesda Press, Silver Spring, 2000, Maryland, p. 256.

125. Both omega-3 and omega-6 fatty acids . . .: Artemis P. Simopoulos, 'The omega-6/
omega-3 fatty acid ratio, genetic variation, and cardiovascular disease', *Asia Pacific*

Journal of Clinical Nutrition, 2008, vol. 17, supplement 1, pp. 131–34, apjcn.nhri. org.tw/server./APJCN/17/s1/131.pdf

125. While humans require essential fatty acids . . .: Bill Lands & Etienne Lamoreaux, 'Using 3–6 differences in essential fatty acids rather than 3/6 ratios gives useful food balance scores', *Nutrition and Metabolism*, 2012, vol. 9, article no. 46, www.ncbi.nlm.nih.gov/pmc/articles/PMC3533819

125. Over the last 150 years . . .: Simopoulous, 'The omega-6/omega-3 fatty acid ratio, genetic variation, and cardiovascular disease'.

125. The typical daily intake of omega-6 . . .: Rachel V. Gow & Joseph R. Hibbeln, 'Omega-3 fatty acid and nutrient deficits in adverse neurodevelopment and childhood behaviors', *Child and Adolescent Psychiatric Clinics of North America*, 2014, vol. 23, no. 3, pp. 555–90.

126. In Australia, canola oil . . .: 'Industry facts and figures', Australian Oilseeds Federation, www.australianoilseeds.com/oilseeds_industry/industry_facts_and_figures

126. Between 1909 and 1999 . . .: Tanya L. Blasbalg et al., 'Changes in consumption of omega-3 and omega-6 fatty acids in the United States during the 20th century', *American Journal of Clinical Nutrition*, 2011, vol. 93, pp. 950–62, ajcn.nutrition. org/content/93/5/950.long

126. While the amount of cottonseed oil . . .: Blasbalg et al., 'Changes in consumption of omega-3 and omega-6 fatty acids in the United States during the 20th century'.

127. Omega-6 and omega-3 content of common seed . . .: SELFNutritionData, 2014, http://nutritiondata.self.com/

127. Omega-6 and omega-3 content of common saturated . . .: Ibid.

127. Omega-3 HUFAs . . .: Anna Wiktorowska-Owczarek et al., 'PUFAs: structures, metabolism and functions', *Advances in Clinical and Experimental Medicine*, 2015, vol. 24, no. 6, pp. 931–41, www.advances.umed.wroc.pl/pdf/2015/24/6/931.pdf; Lucy V. Norling et al., 'Proresolving and cartilage-protective actions of resolving D1 in inflammatory arthritis', *JCI Insight*, 2016, vol. 1, no. 5, article no. e85922, www. ncbi.nlm.nih.gov/pmc/articles/PMC4855303

128. The pro-inflammatory eicosanoids . . .: Bill Lands, 'Omega-3 PUFAs lower the propensity for arachidonic acid cascade overreactions', *BioMed Research International*, 2015, vol. 2015, article no. 285135, www.hindawi.com/journals/bmri/2015/285135

128. Indeed, pharmaceutical companies . . .: Lands & Lamoreaux, 'Using 3–6 differences in essential fatty acids rather than 3/6 ratios gives useful food balance scores'.

128. Aspirin, warfarin, Plavix . . .: Lands, 'Omega-3 PUFAs lower the propensity for arachidonic acid cascade overreactions'.

129. Current research looks to bring back aspirin . . .: A. Masterson, 'Could an aspirin a day keep depression away?', *The Age*, 24 July 2016.

129. In addition to the formation of eicosanoids . . .: Artemis P. Simopoulos, 'An increase in the omega-6/omega-3 fatty acid ratio increases the risk for obesity', *Nutrients*, 2016, vol. 8, no. 3, article no. 128, www.mdpi.com/2072-6643/8/3/128/htm

129. The cannabinoid receptor CB1 . . .: Bill Lands, 'A critique of paradoxes in current advice on dietary lipids', *Progress in Lipid Research*, 2008, vol. 47, no. 2, pp. 77–106.

130. This new partially hydrogenated product . . .: David Schleifer, 'Fear of frying: a brief history of trans fats', *n + 1 magazine*, 21 May 2007, nplusonemag.com/online-only/online-only/fear-frying

131. Keys's idea was supported by . . .: Uffe Ravnskov, *Ignore the Awkward: How the Cholesterol Myths Are Kept Alive*, CreateSpace Independent Publishing Platform, Charleston, South Carolina, 2010, p. 22.

131. For example, deaths from coronary heart . . .: Uffe Ravnskov, *Fat and Cholesterol Are Good for You!*, CreateSpace Independent Publishing Platform, Charleston, South Carolina, 2009, pp. 49–53.

133. In addition, he wanted food processors . . .: Wolfgang Saxon, 'Phil Sokolof, 82, a crusader against cholesterol, is dead', *New York Times*, 17 April 2004, www.nytimes.com/2004/04/17/us/phil-sokolof-82-a-crusader-against-cholesterol-is-dead.html

133. The more alarming finding . . .: Ronald P. Mensink & Martijn B. Katan, 'Effect of dietary trans fatty acids on high-density and low-density lipoprotein cholesterol levels in healthy subjects', *New England Journal of Medicine*, 1990, vol. 323, no. 7, pp. 439–45, http://www.nejm.org/doi/full/10.1056/NEJM199008163230703#t=article

134. The CSPI performed a backflip . . .: David Schleifer, 'How trans fats almost got saturated', *Inform*, January 2014, vol. 25, no. 1, pp. 55–57.

134. In Australia, there are no . . .: Food Standards Australia New Zealand 'Monitoring trans fatty acids', Food Standards Australia New Zealand, January 2015, www.foodstandards.gov.au/science/monitoringnutrients/Pages/Monitoring-of-trans-fatty-acids.aspx

135. Saturated fats make up half . . .: Lands, 'A critique of paradoxes in current advice on dietary lipids'.

135. These HUFAs can be either . . .: Ibid.

136. Deaths from heart disease . . .: Ibid.

137. The researchers found that . . .: Christopher E. Ramsden et al., 'Use of dietary linoleic acid for secondary prevention of coronary heart disease and death: evaluation of recovered data from the Sydney Diet Heart Study and updated meta-analysis', *British Medical Journal*, 2013, vol. 346, article no. e8707, www.bmj.com/content/346/bmj.e8707.long

137. This re-analysis was published . . .: Christopher E. Ramsden et al., 'Re-evaluation of the traditional diet-heart hypothesis: analysis of recovered data from Minnesota Coronary Experiment (1968–73)', *British Medical Journal*, 2016, vol. 353, article no. i1246, www.bmj.com/content/353/bmj.i1246

138. The cannabis plant has been used . . .: Sumner H. Burstein & Robert B. Zurier, 'Cannabinoids, endocannabinoids, and related analogs in inflammation', *American Association of Pharmaceutical Scientists Journal*, 2009, vol. 11, no. 1, article no. 109, www.ncbi.nlm.nih.gov/pmc/articles/PMC2664885

139. Eicosapentaenoic acid from omega-3 . . .: Philip C. Calder & Robert B. Zurier, 'Polyunsaturated fatty acids and rheumatoid arthritis', *Current Opinion in Clinical Nutrition and Metabolic Care*, 2001, vol. 4, no. 2, pp. 115–21.

139. Arabic records from the fifteenth century . . .: Raphael Mechoulam, 'Cannabis – the Israeli perspective', *Journal of Basic and Clinical Physiology and Pharmacology*, 2015, vol. 27, no. 3, pp. 181–87, www.degruyter.com/view/j/jbcpp.2016.27.issue-3/jbcpp-2015-0091/jbcpp-2015-0091.xml

140. The tax was drafted by one Harry Anslinger . . .: Robert Deitch, *Hemp – American History Revisited: The Plant with a Divided History*, Algora, New York, pp. 115, 117

140. The first was CB1 . . .: Guy A. Cabral et al., 'Turning over a new leaf: cannabinoid and endocannabinoid modulation of immune function', *Journal of Neuroimmune Pharmacology*, 2015, vol. 10, pp. 193–203, link.springer.com/article/10.1007/s11481-015-9615-z

141. Both receptors are broadly distributed . . .: Thangesweran Ayakannu et al., 'The endocannabinoid system and sex steroid hormone-dependent cancers', *International Journal of Endocrinology*, 2013, vol. 2013, article no. 259676, www.hindawi.com/journals/ije/2013/259676

141. Research published in 2016 . . .: Judy Lavelle, 'New brain effects behind "runner's high"', *Scientific American*, 8 October 2015, www.scientificamerican.com/article/new-brain-effects-behind-runner-s-high

141. Together, the two cannabinoid receptors . . .: Mechoulam, 'Cannabis – the Israeli perspective'.

142. Once the baby is born . . .: Ester Fride et al., 'The endocannabinoid system during development: emphasis on perinatal events and delayed effects', *Vitamins and Hormones*, 2009, vol. 81, pp.139–58.

142. Balanced endocannabinoid signalling . . .: Mauro Maccarrone et al., 'Endocannabinoid signaling at the periphery: 50 years after THC', *Trends in Pharmacological Sciences*, 2015, vol. 36, no. 5, pp.277–96.

142. According to researchers, dietary fats . . .: Shaan S. Naughton et al., 'Fatty acid modulation of the endocannabinoid system and the effect on food intake and metabolism', *International Journal of Endocrinology*, 2013, vol. 2013, article no. 361895, www.hindawi.com/journals/ije/2013/361895

143. CB1 receptors on neurons . . .: Arnau B. Garcia et al., 'Cannabinoid receptor type-1: breaking the dogmas', *F1000 Research*, 2016, vol. 5, article no. 990, f1000research.com/articles/5-990/v1; S. Ruehle et al., 'The endocannabinoid system in anxiety, fear memory and habituation', *Journal of Psychopharmacology*, vol. 26, no. 1, pp. 23–29, www.ncbi.nlm.nih.gov/pmc/articles/PMC3267552

144. While detailed mechanisms underpinning . . .: Miriam Schneider et al., 'Enhanced functional activity of the cannabinoid type-1 receptor mediates adolescent behaviour', *Journal of Neuroscience*, 2015, vol. 35, no. 41, pp. 13988–75, www.jneurosci.org/content/35/41/13975.long

144. Scientists have also found . . .: Corina O. Bondi et al., 'Adolescent behavior and dopamine availability are uniquely sensitive to dietary omega-3 fatty acid deficiency', *Biological Psychiatry*, 2014, vol. 75, no. 1, pp. 38–46, www.biologicalpsychiatryjournal.com/article/S0006-3223(13)00578-7/fulltext;

Gow & Hibbeln, 'Omega-3 fatty acid and nutrient deficits in adverse neurodevelopment and childhood behaviors'.

144. Researchers from the Avon Longitudinal Study . . .: Joseph R. Hibbeln et al., 'Maternal seafood consumption in pregnancy and neurodevelopmental outcomes in childhood (ALSPAC study): an observational cohort study', *The Lancet*, 2007, vol. 369, no. 9561, pp. 578–85.

144. Moreover, parents of children . . .: Adrian Raine et al., 'Reduction in behavior problems with omega-3 supplementation in children aged 8–16 years: A randomized, double-blind, placebo-controlled, stratified, parallel-group trial', *Journal of Child Psychology and Psychiatry*, 2015, vol. 56, no. 5, pp. 509–20.

145. She credited supplementation . . .: Terry Wahls, 'Minding your mitochondria', TEDx, Iowa City, 2011, www.youtube.com/watch?v=KLjgBLwH3Wc

145. The up-regulation of anandamide . . .: Giuseppe D'Argenio et al., 'Overactivity of the intestinal endocannabinoid system in celiac disease and in methotrexate-treated rats', *Journal of Molecular Medicine*, 2007, vol. 85, no. 5, pp. 523–30.

146. Studies have shown that endocannabinoids . . .: Rupal Pandey et al., 'Endocannabinoids and immune regulation', *Pharmacological Research*, 2009, vol. 60, no. 2, pp. 85–92, www.ncbi.nlm.nih.gov/pmc/articles/PMC3044336

146. Tissue levels of endocannabinoids . . .: Burstein & Zurier, 'Cannabinoids, endocannabinoids, and related analogs in inflammation'.

146. The effect of the endocannabinoid . . .: Maccarrone et al., 'Endocannabinoid signaling at the periphery'.

146. Researchers note that endocannabinoid signalling . . .: Maccarrone et al., 'Endocannabinoid signaling at the periphery'.

147. Elevated endocannabinoid levels . . .: Nicholas V. DiPatrizio et al., 'Endocannabinoid signaling in the gut mediates preference for dietary unsaturated fats', *FASEB Journal*, 2013, vol. 27, no. 6, pp. 2513–20, www.fasebj.org/content/27/6/2513.long

147. Rimonabant, an anti-obesity drug . . .: 'Suicide risk fears over diet pill', BBC News, 15 June 2007, news.bbc.co.uk/2/hi/health/6755665.stm

147. Researchers have hypothesised . . .: DiPatrizio et al., 'Endocannabinoid signaling in the gut mediates preference for dietary unsaturated fats'.

147. Interestingly, endocannabinoids have been . . .: Vincenzo Di Marzo et al., 'Biology of endocannabinoids', in Emmanuel S. Onaivi (ed.), *The Biology of Marijuana: From Gene to Behavior*, Taylor & Francis, London, 2003, pp. 125–174.

148. Apart from health warnings . . .: Artemis P. Simopoulos et al., 'Bellagio report on healthy agriculture, healthy nutrition, healthy people', *Nutrients*, 2013, vol. 5, pp. 411–23, www.ncbi.nlm.nih.gov/pmc/articles/PMC3635202

148. In addition, the American Psychiatric Society . . .: Gow & Hibbeln, 'Omega-3 fatty acid and nutrient deficits in adverse neurodevelopment and childhood behaviors'.

148. In 2014, the American Society for Nutrition . . .: 'Our sustaining partners', American Society for Nutrition, 3 August 2015, www.nutrition.org/our-members/corporate-members/our-sustaining-partners

148. While the paper was mostly . . .: Connie M. Weaver et al., 'Processed foods: contributions to nutrition', scientific statement from the American Society for Nutrition, *American Journal of Clinical Nutrition*, 2014, vol. 99, no. 6, pp. 1525–42, ajcn.nutrition.org/content/99/6/1525.long

6 Can sugar make us sick?

151. Legend has it that in 1598 . . .: John Yudkin, *Pure, White and Deadly: How Sugar Is Killing Us and What We Can Do to Stop it*, Penguin, New York, 2012 (first published 1972), loc 2247 of 3467.

152. Records from the time indicate . . .: Adam Hochschild, *Bury the Chains: The British Struggle to Abolish Slavery*, Pan Books, London, 2012 (first published 2005), p. 34

153. One of the main reasons . . .: Ibid., p. 66.

153. Indeed, the consumption of sugar in Britain . . .: Yudkin, *Pure, White and Deadly*, loc 729 of 3467.

155. It was a British biochemist called . . .: Ibid.

156. He had found, for example . . .: Yudkin, *Pure, White and Deadly*, loc 1663 of 3467.

156. In addition, the aortas of sugar-fed rats . . .: Ibid., loc 1718 of 3467.

156. In human studies, Yudkin found . . .: Ibid., loc 1739 of 3467.

156. But his research . . .: Ibid., loc 1224 of 3467.

157. The introduction noted that more . . .: *Scientific Report of the 2015 Dietary Guidelines Advisory Committee: Advisory Report to the Secretary of Health and Human Services and the Secretary of Agriculture*, USDA and Department of Human and Health Services USA, Washington, DC, 2015, www.health.gov/ dietaryguidelines/2015-scientific-report/PDFs/Scientific-Report-of-the-2015-Dietary-Guidelines-Advisory-Committee.pdf, pp. 1–2.

157. When the official US dietary guidelines . . .: Ferris Jabr, 'Is sugar really toxic? Sifting through the evidence', *Scientific American*, 15 July 2013, blogs.scientificamerican. com/brainwaves/is-sugar-really-toxic-sifting-through-the-evidence

157. At the time of publishing the 2015 guidelines . . .: 'Statistics about diabetes', American Diabetes Association, 1 April 2016, www.diabetes.org/diabetes-basics/statistics

157. The authors also made . . .: *Scientific Report of the 2015 Dietary Guidelines Advisory Committee*, pp. 1–2.

159. The authors speculate that high levels . . .: Kazue Takahashi et al., 'Dietary sugars inhibit biologic functions of the pattern recognition molecule, mannose-binding lectin', *Open Journal of Immunology*, 2011, vol. 1, no. 2, pp. 41–49, www.scirp. org/journal/PaperInformation.aspx?PaperID=7716

160. The Global Burden of Diseases Study . . .: Global Burden of Disease Study 2013 collaborators, 'Global, regional, and national incidence, prevalence, and years lived with disability for 301 acute and chronic diseases and injuries in 188 countries, 1990–2013: a systematic analysis for the Global Burden of Disease Study 2013', *The Lancet*, 2015, vol. 386, no. 9995, pp. 743–800.

160. In some centres, children . . .: Ben Spencer, 'Slap 20% tax on sugary drinks: doctors demand drastic action to fight obesity crisis', *Daily Mail* (Australia), 13 July 2015,

www.dailymail.co.uk/news/article-3158589/Slap-20-tax-sugary-drinks-Doctors-demand-drastic-action-fight-obesity-crisis.html

161. Perhaps most damning . . .: Cristin E. Kearns et al., 'Sugar industry influence on the scientific agenda of the National Institute of Dental Research's 1971 National Caries Program: a historical analysis of internal documents', *PLoS Medicine*, 2015, vol. 12, no. 3, article no. e1001798, journals.plos.org/plosmedicine/article?id=10.1371%2Fjournal.pmed.1001798

161. He has also been credited . . .: Fredric B. Kraemer & Henry N. Ginsberg, 'Gerald M. Reaven, MD: demonstration of the central role of insulin resistance in type 2 diabetes and cardiovascular disease', *Diabetes Care*, 2014, vol. 37, no. 5, pp. 1178–81, care.diabetesjournals.org/content/37/5/1178.long

162. Today the official metabolic syndrome . . .: K.G.M.M. Alberti et al. 'Harmonizing the metabolic syndrome: a joint interim statement of the International Diabetes Federation Task Force on Epidemiology and Prevention; National Heart, Lung, and Blood Institute; American Heart Association; World Heart Federation; International Atherosclerosis Society; and International Association for the Study of Obesity', *Circulation*, 2009, vol. 120, no. 16, pp. 1640–45, circ.ahajournals.org/content/120/16/1640.long

162. Reaven also noted that simply . . .: Louise Morrin, 'An interview with Gerald Reaven: syndrome X: the risks of insulin resistance', *Canadian Association of Cardiovascular Prevention and Rehabilitation Newsletter*, September 2000, www.cacpr.ca/information_for_public/archived_issues/2000s/0009Reaven.pdf

162. Although not part of its current . . .: Rajesh Tota-Maharaj et al. 'A practical approach to the metabolic syndrome: review of current concepts and management', *Current Opinion in Cardiology*, 2010, vol. 25, no. 5, pp. 502–12.

162. Their own investigation detected . . .: Quanhe Yang et al., 'Added sugar intake and cardiovascular diseases mortality among US adults', *JAMA Internal Medicine*, 2014, vol. 174, no. 4, pp. 516–24, archinte.jamanetwork.com/article.aspx?articleid=1819573

164. In animal experiments, feeding . . .: Luc Tappy, 'Q&A: "Toxic" effects of sugar: should we be afraid of fructose?' *BMC Biology*, 2012, vol. 10, article no. 42, bmcbiol.biomedcentral.com/articles/10.1186/1741-7007-10-42

164. In addition, fructose is the only . . .: Stephanie Nguyen et al., 'Sugar-sweetened beverages, serum uric acid, and blood pressure in adolescents', *Journal of Pediatrics*, 2009, vol. 154, no. 6, pp. 807–13, www.ncbi.nlm.nih.gov/pmc/articles/PMC2727470

164. In his 2015 book *Sugar Crush* . . .: Richard P. Jacoby & Raquel Baldelomar, *Sugar Crush: How to Reduce Inflammation, Reverse Nerve Damage, and Reclaim Good Health*, HarperCollins, New York, 2015.

165. Then come the ulcers . . .: Ibid., p. 101.

165. Dr Jacoby's book makes sober . . .: Ibid., p. 96.

166. Further studies on diabetic ulcers . . .: Atanu Biswas et al., 'Use of sugar on the healing of diabetic ulcers: a review', *Journal of Diabetes Science and Technology*, 2010, vol. 4, no. 5, pp. 1139–45, dst.sagepub.com/content/4/5/1139.long

167. The researchers also calculated . . .: Cindy W. Leung et al., 'Soda and cell aging: associations between sugar-sweetened beverage consumption and leukocyte telomere length in healthy adults from the National Health and Nutrition Examination Surveys', *American Journal of Public Health*, 2014, vol. 104, no. 12, pp. 2425–31.

167. To make things worse . . .: Philip C. Haycock et al., 'Leukocyte telomere length and risk of cardiovascular disease: systematic and meta-analysis', *British Medical Journal*, 2014; vol. 349, article no. g4227, www.bmj.com/content/349/bmj.g4227

167. A 2005 study also revealed . . .: A.M. Valdes et al., 'Obesity, cigarette smoking, and telomere length in women', *The Lancet*, 2005, vol. 366, no. 9486, pp. 662–64.

168. In addition, Indigenous women . . .: Australian Institute of Health and Welfare, *Cancer in Aboriginal and Torres Strait Islander Peoples of Australia: An Overview*, Australian Government, Canberra, 2013, p. xi.

168. That Indigenous Australians consume . . .: 'Diabetes expert wants Coke out of communities', ABC News, 2 April 2010, www.abc.net.au/news/2010–04–02/diabetes-expert-wants-coke-out-of-communities/389680?site=alicesprings

168. According to a 2007 report . . .: World Cancer Research Fund & American Institute for Cancer Research, *Food, Nutrition, Physical Activity and the Prevention of Cancer: a Global Perspective*, AICR, Washington, DC, 2007, p. 374, www.dietandcancerreport.org/cancer_resource_center/downloads/chapters/chapter_12.pdf

168. And finally, elevated levels of sex steroid . . .: Ibid., p.39.

168. The World Cancer Research Fund notes . . .: 'Our Cancer Prevention Recommendations', World Cancer Research International, accessed September 2016, http://wcrf.org/int/research-we-fund/our-cancer-prevention-recommendations

169. [Diagram]: 'Food, Nutrition, Physical Activity, and the Prevention of Cancer: a Global Perspective', World Cancer Research Fund & American Institute for Cancer Research, Washington DC, 2007, http://www.aicr.org/assets/docs/pdf/reports/Second_Expert_Report.pdf

170. In laboratory studies, glucose . . .: Aaron Lerner & Torsten Matthias, 'Changes in intestinal tight junction permeability associated with industrial food additives explain the rising incidence of autoimmune disease', *Autoimmunity Reviews*, 2015, vol. 14, no. 6, pp. 479–89, www.sciencedirect.com/science/article/pii/S1568997215000245

171. Over the last twenty years . . .: Meagan Phelan, 'Science: researchers hunt origin of an enigmatic kidney disease', American Association for Advancement of Science, 10 April 2014, www.aaas.org/news/science-researchers-hunt-origin-enigmatic-kidney-disease

171. Seven out of ten men there . . .: Ariadne Ellsworth, 'Sickly sweet: the sugar cane industry and kidney disease', *Brown Political Review*, 7 June 2014, www.brownpoliticalreview.org/2014/06/sickly-sweet-the-link-between-the-sugar-cane-industry-and-chronic-kidney-disease-of-unknown-origin

171. While researchers have debated . . .: Channa Jayasumana et al., 'Glyphosate, hard water and nephrotoxic metals: are they the culprits behind the epidemic of

chronic kidney disease of unknown etiology in Sri Lanka?', *International Journal of Environmental Research and Public Health*, 2014, vol. 11, no. 2, pp. 2125–47, www.ncbi.nlm.nih.gov/pmc/articles/PMC3945589

172. 'Every family here . . .': Nina Lakhani, 'Nicaraguans demand action over illness killing thousands of sugar cane workers', *The Guardian*, 16 February 2015, www.theguardian.com/world/2015/feb/16/-sp-nicaragua-kidney-disease-killing-sugar-cane-workers

172. In a further attempt to distance . . .: Ibid.

173. The government of President José Ortega . . .: Ibid.

7 Can wheat make us sick

175. In 1979 *Washington Post* . . .: Dan Morgan, *The Merchants of Grain: The Power and Profits of the Five Giant Companies at the Centre of the World's Food Supply*, Viking, New York, 1979.

176. A June 2013 consumer survey . . .: 'U.S. consumers' reasons for eating gluten-free foods 2013', Statista, www.statista.com/statistics/304324/us-consumers-reasons-for-eating-gluten-free-food

177. A grain of wheat consists of three parts . . .: Peter R. Shewry, 'Wheat', *Journal of Experimental Botany*, 2009, vol. 60, no. 6, pp. 1537–53, jxb.oxfordjournals.org/content/60/6/1537.long

177. The prevalence of CD . . .: S. Lohi et al., 'Increasing prevalence of coeliac disease over time', Alimentary Pharmacology and Therapeutics, 2007, vol. 26, no. 9, pp. 1217–25, onlinelibrary.wiley.com/doi/10.1111/j.1365-2036.2007.03502.x/full; Hetty C. van den Broek et al., 'Presence of celiac disease epitopes in modern and old hexaploid wheat varieties: wheat breeding may have contributed to increased prevalence of celiac disease', *Theoretical and Applied Genetics*, 2010, vol. 121, no. 8, pp. 1527–39, link.springer.com/article/10.1007%2Fs00122-010-1408-4

178. Another gluten-related condition . . .: Francesco Tovoli et al., 'Clinical and diagnostic aspects of gluten related disorders', *World Journal of Clinical Cases*, 2015, vol. 3, no. 3, pp. 275–84, ncbi.nlm.nih.gov/pmc/articles/PMC4360499

178. It's most often found . . .: Ibid.

178. Genes for proteins at the dermal–epidermal junction . . .: M. Dolcino et al., 'Gene expression profiling in dermatitis herpetiformis skin lesions', *Clinical and Developmental Immunology*, 2012, vol. 2012, article no. 198956, www.hindawi.com/journals/jir/2012/198956

178. Wheat allergy includes four main conditions . . .: Tovoli et al., 'Clinical and diagnostic aspects of gluten related disorders'.

179. In addition to coeliac disease . . .: Jonas F. Ludvigsson et al., 'The Oslo definitions for coeliac disease and related terms', *Gut*, 2013, vol. 62, no. 1, pp. 43–52, gut.bmj.com/content/62/1/43.long; Antonio Carroccio et al., 'Non-celiac wheat sensitivity diagnosed by double-blind placebo-controlled challenge: exploring a new clinical entity', *American Journal of Gastroenterology*, 2012, vol. 107, pp.1898–906.

179. NCGS differs from coeliac disease . . .: Rubio-Tapia et al., 'ACG clinical guidelines: diagnosis and management of celiac disease'.

179. Researchers first raised the possibility . . .: B.T. Cooper et al., 'Gluten-sensitive diarrhea without evidence of celiac disease', *Gastroenterology*, 1980, vol. 79, no. 5, pp. 801–806.

179. These symptoms include . . .: Umberto Volta et al., 'An Italian prospective multicenter survey on patients suspected of having non-celiac gluten sensitivity', *BMC Medicine*, 2014, vol. 12, article no. 85, bmcmedicine.biomedcentral.com/articles/10.1186/1741-7015-12-85

180. Pasquale Mansueto and his colleagues . . .: Pasquale Mansueto et al., 'Non-celiac gluten sensitivity: literature review', *Journal of the American College of Nutrition*, 2014, vol. 33, no. 1, pp. 39–54.

180. This is unacceptable given the condition . . .: Ludvigsson et al., 'The Oslo definitions for coeliac disease and related terms'.

180. 'Diagnosis of non-coeliac gluten sensitivity . . .': Carlo Catassi et al., 'Diagnosis of non-celiac gluten sensitivity (NCGS): the Salerno Experts' Criteria', *Nutrients*, 2015, vol. 7, no. 6, pp. 4966–77, www.ncbi.nlm.nih.gov/pmc/articles/PMC4488826

181. Once this occurs, these 'leaks' . . .: Alessio Fasano, 'Zonulin, regulation of tight junctions, and autoimmune disease', *Annals of the New York Academy of Sciences*, 2012, vol. 1258, no. 1, pp. 25–33, ncbi.nlm.nih.gov/pmc/articles/PMC3384703

181. In the late 1980s . . .:Alessio Fasano, 'Surprises from celiac disease', *Scientific American*, August 2009, vol. 301, pp. 54–61.

181. Fasano is famous for his maxim . . .: Alessio Fasano with Susie Flaherty, *Gluten Freedom: The Nation's Leading Expert Offers the Essential Guide to a Healthy, Gluten Free Lifestyle*, Turner Publishing, New York, 2014, loc 1191 of 5437.

182. It has since been shown that . . .: Fasano, 'Surprises from celiac disease'.

182. In his many interviews and presentations . . .: Justin Hollon et al., 'Effect of gliadin on permeability of intestinal biopsy explants from celiac disease patients and patients with non-celiac gluten sensitivity', *Nutrients*, 2015, vol. 7, no. 3, pp. 1565–76, mdpi.com/2072-6643/7/3/1565/htm

183. In addition, Fasano has often . . .: Fasano, 'Surprises from celiac disease'.

184. Professor Fasano writes in his 2014 book . . .: Fasano with Flaherty, *Gluten Freedom*, loc 1587–1859 of 5437.

184. In addition, a 2006 literature review . . .: A.E. Kalaydjian et al., 'The gluten connection: the association between schizophrenia and celiac disease', *Acta Psychiatrica Scandinavica*, 2006, vol. 113, no. 2, pp. 82–90.

184. The researchers noted . . .: F.C. Dohan et al., 'Is schizophrenia rare if grain is rare?', *Biological Psychiatry*, 1984, vol. 19, no. 3, pp. 385–99.

185. The paper reports that even . . .: Elena Lionetti et al., 'Gluten psychosis: confirmation of a new clinical entity', *Nutrients*, 2015, vol. 7, no. 7, pp. 5532–39, www.mdpi.com/2072-6643/7/7/5235/htm

185. Recent studies have suggested . . .: B. Zanini et al. '"Non celiac gluten sensitivity" (NCGS) is uncommon in patients spontaneously adhering to gluten free diet

(GFD) and is outnumbered by "FODMAPs sensitivity"', *Gut*, 2014, vol. 63, article no. A260, gut.bmj.com/content/63/Suppl_1/A260.1.full.pdf+html; Jessica R. Biesiekierski et al., 'No effects of gluten in patients with self-reported non-celiac gluten sensitivity after dietary reduction of fermentable, poorly absorbed short chain carbohydrates', *Gastroenterology*, 2013, vol. 145, no. 2, pp. 320–28, www.gastrojournal.org/article/S0016-5085(13)00702-6/fulltext

186. According to the USDA . . .: SELFNutritionData, http://nutritiondata.self.com/

187. Indeed, studies suggest a dysregulated . . .: Natalia Battista et al., 'Altered expression of type-1 and type-2 cannabinoid receptors in celiac disease', *PLoS One*, 2013, vol. 8, no. 4, journals.plos.org/plosone/article?id=10.1371/journal.pone.0062078

187. Lipopolysaccharides are known . . .: Karin de Punder & Leo Pruimboom, 'Stress induces endotoxemia and low-grade inflammation by increasing barrier permeability', *Frontiers in Immunology*, 2015, vol. 6, article no. 223, journal. frontiersin.org/article/10.3389/fimmu.2015.00223/full

187. Elevated blood levels of major . . .: Michael Maes et al., 'The gut-brain barrier in major depression: intestinal mucosal dysfunction with an increased translocation of LPS from gram negative enterobacteria (leaky gut) plays a role in the inflammatory pathophysiology of depression', *Neuroendocrinology Letters*, 2008, vol. 29, no. 1, p. 120, at jeffreydachmd.com/wp-content/uploads/2013/03/Leaky-gut-brain-barrier-in-major-depression-LPS-from-gram-negative-bacteria-Michael-Maes-Neuroendocrinology-2008.pdf

187. While higher endotoxin levels . . .: de Punder & Pruimboom, 'Stress induces endotoxemia and low-grade inflammation by increasing barrier permeability'.

188. One study conducted in India . . .: B. Jayashree et al., 'Increased circulatory levels of lipopolysaccharide (LPS) and zonulin signify novel biomarkers of proinflammation in patients with type 2 diabetes', *Molecular Cell Biochemistry*, 2014, vol. 388, nos 1–2, pp. 203–10.

188. The authors expressed alarm . . .: S. Sadeghi et al., 'Dietary lipids modify the cytokine response to bacterial lipopolysaccharide in mice', *Immunology*, 1999, vol. 96, no. 3, pp. 404–10, https://www.ncbi.nlm.nih.gov/pmc/articles/PMC2326770/

188. They are also understood to play a role . . .: D. Schuppan & V. Zevallos, 'Wheat amylase trypsin inhibitors as nutritional activators of innate immunity', *Digestive Diseases*, 2015, vol. 33, no. 2, pp. 260–63.

188. The ATI content of wheat . . .: Yvonne Junker et al., 'Wheat amylase trypsin inhibitors drive intestinal inflammation via activation of toll-like receptor 4', *Journal of Experimental Medicine*, 2012, vol. 209, no. 13, pp. 2395–408, jem. rupress.org/content/209/13/2395.long

189. Wheatgerm agglutinin (WGA) is a lectin . . .: Ilka M. Vasconcelos & José T.A. Oliveira, 'Antinutritional properties of plant lectins', *Toxicon*, 2004, vol. 44, no. 4, pp. 385–403.

189. Lectins (from the Latin . . .: Els J.M. Van Damme et al., *Handbook of Plant Lectins: Properties and Biomedical Applications*, John Wiley & Sons, Chichester, 1998 p. 31.

189. This means that lectins . . .: Aphichart Karnchanatat, 'Antimicrobial activity of lectins from plants', in Varaprasad Bobbarala (ed.), *Antimicrobial Agents*,

InTech, Rijeka, Croatia, 2012, www.intechopen.com/books/antimicrobial-agents/antimicrobial-activity-of-lectins-from-antimicrobial-activity-of-lectins-from-plants

189. Indeed, according to one research group . . .: Ajit Varki & Hudson H. Freeze, 'Glycans in acquired human diseases', and Ajit Varki et al., 'Glycosylation changes in cancer', in Ajit Varki et al. (eds), *Essentials of Glycobiology*, 2nd edn, Cold Spring Harbor Laboratory Press, Cold Spring Harbor, New York, 2009, www.ncbi.nlm.nih.gov/books/NBK1963

189. WGA has also been linked . . .: Peter J. D'Adamo, *Fundamentals of Generative Medicine*, Drum Hill Publishing, Wilton Connecticut, p. 707, www.dadamo.com/pdf/dadamo_fgmtxt_glycomics.pdf

189. The role that lectins play . . .: Gianni Vandenborre et al., 'Plant lectins as defense proteins against phytophagous insects', *Phytochemistry*, 2011, vol. 72, no. 13, pp. 1538–50.

189. Not all plant lectins are considered . . .: Ibid.

189. According to Arpad Pusztai . . .: A. Pusztai, 'Dietary lectins are metabolic signals for the gut and modulate immune and hormonal functions', *European Journal of Clinical Nutrition*, vol. 47, no. 10, pp. 691–99.

190. After a decades-long career . . .: A. Pusztai et al., 'Antinutritive effects of wheat-germ agglutinin and other N-acetylglucosamine-specific lectins', *British Journal Nutrition*, 1993, vol. 70, no. 1, pp. 313–21.

190. In 1999, the eminent allergist . . .: David L.J. Freed, 'Do dietary lectins cause disease?', *British Medical Journal*, 1999, vol. 318, no. 7190, pp. 1023–24, www.ncbi.nlm.nih.gov/pmc/articles/PMC1115436

190. Freed noted that wheat . . .: Loren Cordain et al., 'Modulation of immune function by dietary lectins in rheumatoid arthritis', *British Journal of Nutrition*, 2000, vol. 83, no. 3, pp. 207–17.

190. Anecdotally, sufferers of rheumatoid arthritis . . .: D'Adamo, *Fundamentals of Generative Medicine*.

191. The blood-type diet forbids . . .: Peter J. D'Adamo, *Eat Right 4 Your Type*, Arrow Books, London, 2001.

191. One major issue concerning . . .: Jingzhu Wang et al., 'ABO genotype, "blood-type" diet and cardiometabolic risk factors', *PLoS One*, 2014, vol. 9, no. 1, article no. e84749, https://www.ncbi.nlm.nih.gov/pmc/articles/PMC3893150/#pone.0084749.s002

191. While a 2014 article . . .: Vincent J. van Buul & Fred J.P.H. Brouns, 'Health effects of wheat lectins: a review', *Journal of Cereal Science*, 2014, vol. 59, no. 2, pp. 112–17; Karin de Punder & Leo Pruimboon, 'The dietary intake of wheat and other cereal grains and their role in inflammation', *Nutrients*, 2013, vol. 5, no. 3, pp. 771–87, www.mdpi.com/2072-6643/5/3/771

191. Wheat contains phytic acid . . .: Karen H.C. Lim et al., 'Iron and zinc nutrition in the economically-developed world: a review', *Nutrients*, 2013, vol. 5, no. 8, pp. 3184–211, www.mdpi.com/2072-6643/5/8/3184/htm

192. Iron deficiency is the most common . . .: Sant-Rayn Pasricha et al., 'Control of iron deficiency anemia in low- and middle-income countries', *Blood*, 2013, vol. 121, no. 14, pp. 2607–17, www.bloodjournal.org/content/121/14/2607.long

192. Iron is also required . . .: Antigone Kouris, *Food Sources of Nutrients: A Ready Reckoner of Macronutrients, Micronutrients and Phytonutrients*, Lulu.com, Raleigh, North Carolina, 2011, p. 15; Osiecki, *The Nutrient Bible*, pp. 179–80.

193. According to a nutrition survey . . .: Taylor C. Wallace et al., 'Calcium and vitamin D disparities are related to gender, age, race, household income level, and weight classification but not vegetarian status in the United States: analysis of the NHANES 2001–2008 data set', *Journal of the American College of Nutrition*, 2013, vol. 32, no. 5, pp. 321–30.

193. Magnesium deficiency potentially . . .: Osiecki, *The Nutrient Bible*, pp. 182–83.

194. It regulates body temperature . . .: Kouris, *Food Sources of Nutrients*, p. 16.

194. He was involved, for example . . .: Megan Scudellari, 'Mutagens and multivitamins', *The Scientist*, 1 June 2014, www.the-scientist.com/?articles.view/articleNo/40054/title/Mutagens-and-Multivitamins

194. Zinc is required for more than . . .: Emily Ho & Bruce N. Ames, 'Low intracellular zinc induces oxidative DNA damage, disrupts p53, NFκB, and AP1 DNA binding, and affects DNA repair in a rat glioma cell line', *Proceedings of the National Academy of Sciences*, 2002, vol. 99, no. 26, pp. 16770–75, www.ncbi.nlm.nih.gov/pmc/articles/PMC139219

194. Ames's research suggests . . .: Ibid.

195. Zinc deficiency is associated . . .: Nriagu, 'Zinc deficiency in human health'; Ananda S. Prasad, 'Zinc in human health: effect of zinc on immune cells', *Molecular Medicine*, 2008, vol. 14, nos 5–6, pp. 353–57, www.ncbi.nlm.nih.gov/pmc/articles/PMC2277319

195. While Ames admits to a lack . . .: Scudellari, 'Mutagens and multivitamins'.

195. One of the best known books . . .: William Davis, *Wheat Belly: Lose the Wheat, Lose the Weight, and Find Your Path Back to Health*, Rodale, New York, 2011.

196. The group that consumed the Khorasan products . . .: Anne Whittaker et al., 'An organic khorasan wheat-based replacement diet improves risk profile of patients with acute coronary syndrome: a randomised crossover trial', *Nutrients*, 2015, vol. 7, no. 5, pp. 3401–15

197. No such effects were observed . . .: Francesco Sofi et al., 'Characterisation of khorasan wheat (Kamut) and impact of a replacement diet on cardiovascular risk factors: cross-over dietary intervention study', *European Journal of Clinical Nutrition*, 2013, vol. 67, pp. 190–95, www.nature.com/ejcn/journal/v67/n2/full/ejcn2012206a.html

197. Symptoms such as abdominal pain . . .: Francesco Sofi et al., 'Effect of *Triticum turgidum* subsp. *turanicum* wheat on irritable bowel syndrome: a double-blinded randomized dietary intervention trial', *British Journal of Nutrition*, 2014, vol. 111, no. 11, pp. 1992–99, https://www.ncbi.nlm.nih.gov/pubmed/24521561

198. 'Diabetes is a disease of carbohydrate intolerance . . .': Richard D. Feinman, *The World Turned Upside Down: The Second Low-carbohydrate Revolution*, NMS Press, Snohomish, Washington, 2014, loc 2733 of 5850.

199. The authors (26 medical specialists . . .: Richard D. Feinman et al., 'Dietary carbohydrate restriction as the first approach in diabetes management: critical review and evidence base', *Nutrition*, 2015, vol. 31, no. 1, pp. 1–13, www.nutritionjrnl.com/article/S0899-9007(14)00332-3/fulltext

201. Hallberg notes substantial cost savings . . .: Sarah Hallberg & Wayne Campbell, 'Retrospective analysis of metabolic control in type 2 diabetes with American Diabetes Association recommendations compared with carbohydrate restriction', *Journal of Clinical Lipidology*, 2015, vol. 9, no. 3, p. 240, www.lipidjournal.com/article/S1933-2874(15)00113-0/abstract

202. He credits the low-carbohydrate diet . . .: Richard Bernstein speaking at the Nutrition and Metabolism Society Meeting, 8 May 2010, www.youtube.com/watch?v=RVYGjETjHPA

205. So impressed was he with . . .: William Banting, 'Letter on Corpulence', 3rd edition, *Internet Archive*, 1864, https://archive.org/details/letteroncorpulen00bant

205. After all, the low-fat, high-carbohydrate diet . . .: Surender K. Arora & Samy I. McFarlane, 'The case for low carbohydrate diets in diabetes management', *Nutrition and Metabolism*, 2005, vol. 2, article no. 16, www.ncbi.nlm.nih.gov/pmc/articles/PMC1188071

205. Until recently, the reason for . . .: 'Welcome to OxHA.org', Oxford Health Alliance, 2015, www.oxha.org

207. She also notes that by 2030 . . .: Pamela Dyson, 'Low carbohydrate diets and type 2 diabetes: what is the latest evidence?', *Diabetes Therapy*, 2015, vol. 6, no. 4, pp. 411–24, www.ncbi.nlm.nih.gov/pmc/articles/PMC4674467

207. While Dyson declared no conflict . . .: Pamela Dyson, 'Erratum to: Low carbohydrate diets and type 2 diabetes: what is the latest evidence?', *Diabetes Therapy*, 2015, vol. 6, no. 4, p. 649, www.ncbi.nlm.nih.gov/pmc/articles/PMC4674465

207. Other funding partners include . . .: 'Supporting OxHA', The Oxford Health Alliance website, 2015, www.oxha.org/about-us/supporting-oxha; 'Diabetes Australia Corporate Partners', Diabetes Australia, 2015, www.diabetesaustralia.com.au/corporate-partners; 'Corporate Partnerships', Stroke Foundation, 2016, strokefoundation.com.au/donate/corporate-partnerships; 'Funding partners', Heart Foundation (Australia), www.heartfoundation.org.au/research/funding-partners

208. In a later paper published by Dyson . . .: Pamela Dyson, 'Saturated fat and Type 2 Diabetes: where do we stand?', *Diabetic Medicine*, 27 June 2016, http://onlinelibrary.wiley.com/doi/10.1111/dme.13176/abstract

209. The researchers also noted . . .: Faidah Amin & Anwar H. Gilani, 'Fiber-free white flour with fructose offers a better model of metabolic syndrome', *Lipids in Health and Disease*, 2013, vol. 12, article no. 44, lipidworld.biomedcentral.com/articles/10.1186/1476-511X-12-44

209. The most recent Australian Health Survey . . .: Australian Bureau of Statistics, '4364.0.55.007 – Australian Health Survey: nutrition first results – foods and nutrients, 2011–2012: carbohydrate', ABS, 9 May 2014, www.abs.gov.au/ausstats/abs@.nsf/Lookup/by Subject/4364.0.55.007~2011–12~Main

Features~Carbohydrate~705; Feinman, et. al., 'Dietary carbohydrate restriction as the first approach in diabetes management: critical review and evidence base'.

209. The Dietitians Association of Australia . . .: Dietitians Association of Australia, 'Low carbohydrate, high fat diets for diabetes', media release, DAA, August 2015, daa.asn.au/for-the-media/hot-topics-in-nutrition/low-carbohydrate-high-fat-diets-for-diabetes

210. It's curious, then, that independent . . .: Ibid.

210. In 2013 the sales of diabetes drugs . . .: Ed Silverman, 'Dubious ties and surrogate markers expand the market for diabetes drugs', *Wall Street Journal*, 22 December 2014, blogs.wsj.com/pharmalot/2014/12/22/dubious-ties-and-surrogate-markers-expand-the-market-for-diabetes-drugs

210. One of the experts the journalists interviewed . . .: Mary O'Hara & Pamela Duncan, 'Why "big pharma" stopped searching for the next Prozac', *The Guardian*, 27 January 2016, www.theguardian.com/society/2016/jan/27/prozac-next-psychiatric-wonder-drug-research-medicine-mental-illness

211. Yudkin reveals that the BNF . . .: Yudkin, *Pure, White and Deadly*, loc 3038 of 3467.

211. To counter the issue . . .: Yudkin, *Pure, White and Deadly*, loc 3038 of 3467.

212. This phenomenon, known as pseudoscepticism . . .: Michael Shermer, 'What can be done about pseudoskepticism? Just because we don't know everything doesn't mean we know nothing', *Scientific American*, vol. 312, no. 3, 17 February 2015, www.scientificamerican.com/article/what-can-be-done-about-pseudoskepticism

213. When evidence is produced . . .: Shermer, 'What can be done about pseudoskepticism?'.

213. The art and practice of pseudoscepticism . . .: Naomi Oreskes & Erik M. Conway, *Merchants of Doubt: How a Handful of Scientists Obscured the Truth on Issues from Tobacco Smoke to Global Warming*, Bloomsbury, London, 2010.

213. Yudkin's unyielding belief . . .: Yudkin, *Pure, White and Deadly*, loc 2968 of 3467.

8 The diet wars

215. Only this time she was dealing . . .: Joseph Schwartz, 'U.S. Media Publishers and Publications – Ranked for July 2016', *Market Trends*, SimilarWeb, 14 August 2016, https://www.similarweb.com/blog/us-media-publishers-july-2016

216. In his 2013 book *The End of Power* . . .: Moisés Naím, *The End of Power: From Boardrooms to Battlefields and Churches to States, Why Being in Charge Isn't What it Used to Be*, Basic Books, New York, 2013.

218. In 2013, nutritionist Bill Shrapnel . . .: Angus Holland, 'Sweet assassin', *Sydney Morning Herald*, 30 January 2013, http://www.smh.com.au/lifestyle/diet-and-fitness/sweet-assassin-20130121-2d2o7.html

218. Shrapnel was one of fourteen health experts . . .: Journey staff, 'Our commitment to transparency: list of health professionals and scientific experts', Coca-Cola Journey, 14 March 2016, transparency.coca-colajourney.com.au/health-professionals-and-scientific-experts

218. Shrapnel runs a nutrition blog . . .: Bill Shrapnel, The Sceptical Nutritionist: The Science and Ideology of Healthy Eating, scepticalnutritionist.com.au

219. The peer-reviewed paper . . .: Alan W. Barclay & Jennie Brand-Miller, 'The Australian paradox: a substantial decline in sugars intake over the same timeframe that overweight and obesity has increased', *Nutrition*, 2011, vol. 3, no. 4, pp. 491–504, www.ncbi.nlm.nih.gov/pmc/articles/PMC3257688

219. Based upon these conclusions . . .: 'The Australian Beverages Council submission to: NHMRC Australian Dietary Guidelines', 28 February 2012, p. 37, www.abc.net.au/cm/lb/5251976/data/bev-sub-to-nhmrc-data.pdf

220. The study was also used . . .: Australian Beverages Council, 'Why a soft drinks tax is not the answer', VicHealth Citizen's Jury on Obesity, 25 August 2015, collab. vichealth.vic.gov.au/cjo/b/submissions/archive/2015/08/25/australian-beverage-council-why-a-soft-drinks-tax-is-not-the-answer

220. The Australian Beverages Council along with . . .: Community Portal, VicHealth, collab.vichealth.vic.gov.au/cjo/p/about

220. One person who took exception . . .: Rory Robertson, The Australian Paradox: A Critical Analysis (website), www.australianparadox.com

220. 'not-for-profit University of Sydney spin-off company': 'Meet our people: Professor Jennie Brand-Miller', Sydney University, sydney.edu.au/recruitment/our-people

221. Alan Barclay was also named in 2016 . . .: Journey staff, 'List of health professionals and scientific experts', Coca-Cola Journey, 14 March 2016, transparency.coca-colajourney.com.au/health-professionals-and-scientific-experts

221. The investigation did not uphold . . .Robert Clark, 'Initial inquiry report: complaint by Mr. Rory Robertson against Professor Jennie Brand-Miller and Dr Alan Barclay', *The University of Sydney*, 26 June 2014, https://ses.library.usyd.edu.au//bitstream/2123/15705/2/australian-paradox-report-redacted.pdf

221. In an interview . . .: Mark Metherell, 'Research causes stir over sugar's role in obesity', *Sydney Morning Herald*, 31 March 2012, www.smh.com.au/national/health/research-causes-stir-over-sugars-role-in-obesity-20120330-1w3e5.html

222. Prominent dietitian Rosemary Stanton . . .: Sarah Whyte, 'Affluent develop taste for gluten-free', *Sydney Morning Herald*, 20 July 2013, www.smh.com.au/national/affluent-develop-taste-for-glutenfree-20130719-2q9rz.html

222. (It's worth noting here . . .: 'Contributors', Grains & Legumes Nutrition Council, www.glnc.org.au/about-us/contributors

222. In April 2015, the GLNC . . .: Sue Dunlevy, 'Paleo diet and gluten free fad behind 30 per cent fall in grain consumption in three years', News Limited, 30 April 2015, http://www.news.com.au/lifestyle/health/diet/paleo-diet-and-gluten-free-fad-behind-30-per-cent-fall-in-grain-consumption-in-three-years/news-story/7348884ab3f1c4b4d338f712ac17930c

222. Another code red was issued . . .: Ibid.

223. In July 2014, the DAA . . .: DAA, 'Don't go the Paleo way', July 2014, http://www.medianet.com.au/releases/release-details/?id=806638

223. Another sponsor, US-owned Campbell Soup . . .: Carly Weeks, 'Campbell's adding salt back to its soups', *Globe and Mail*, 14 July 2011, www.theglobeandmail.com/life/health-and-fitness/campbells-adding-salt-back-to-its-soups/article587037

223. The 'dangerous' claims were followed . . .: Stacy Farrar, 'Australia, I implore you, we must not give up on bread', *Daily Telegraph*, 30 April 2015, www.dailytelegraph.com.au/rendezview/australia-i-implore-you-we-must-not-give-up-on-bread/story-fnpug1jf-1227328959412

224. And as we have seen, when nutrition . . .: Kirby, 'Kerin O'Dea: improving the health of indigenous Australians'.

224. In 2015, it issued a 'hot topic' release . . .: DAA, 'Hot topics in nutrition', July 2015, http://web.archive.org/web/20150730002907/http://daa.asn.au/for-the-media/hot-topics-in-nutrition

224. Dr Sikaris's observation . . .: Julia Medew, 'Fatty liver disease: the frightening epidemic affecting one in three Australians', *The Age*, 14 December 2015, www.smh.com.au/national/fatty-liver-disease-the-frightening-epidemic-affecting-one-in-three-australians-20151213-glmgbw.html

225. Contrast the actions of the DAA . . .: Best Health, 'News: Heart and Stroke Foundation ends Health Check program', http://www.besthealthmag.ca/blog-post/news-heart-and-stroke-foundation-ends-health-check-program/

225. Having terminated the program . . .: Heart & Stroke Foundation of Canada, 'Health check exit'; Heart & Stroke Foundation of Canada, 'Sugar, heart disease and stroke', position statement, September 2014, www.heartandstroke.com/site/c.ikIQLcMWJtE/b.9201361/k.47CB/Sugar_heart_disease_and_stroke.htm

226. Indeed, consumers obtained their nutritional information . . .: Institute for the Future, 'The future of health and wellness in food retailing: results from a national survey', IFTF, Palo Alto, California, April 2008, p. 16, http://www.iftf.org/our-work/global-landscape/global-food-outlook/the-future-of-health-wellness-in-food-retailing/

226. In 2015, Coca-Cola published . . .: Journey staff, 'List of health professionals and scientific experts', Coca-Cola Journey.

226. An analysis by the Ninjas for Health . . .: Kyle Pfister, 'The new faces of Coke', Ninjas for Health, 20 September 2015, medium.com/the-death-of-the-sugar-industry/the-new-faces-of-coke-62314047160f

226. Of the 27 named, thirteen . . .: 'Our investments in health and wellbeing research and partnerships – individuals', Coca-Cola Great Britain, 18 December 2015, www.coca-cola.co.uk/list-of-health-professionals-and-scientific-experts

229. The number of allergy sufferers . . .: Australian Society of Clinical Immunology and Allergy, 'Allergy and immune diseases in Australia (AIDA) report 2013', ASCIA, Sydney, 2013, p. 4, www.allergy.org.au/images/stories/reports/ASCIA_AIDA_Report_2013.pdf

229. Almost 20 per cent of Australians . . .: ASCIA, 'Allergy and immune diseases in Australia (AIDA) report 2013', p. 2.

230. Of particular concern is . . .: ASCIA, 'Allergy and immune diseases in Australia (AIDA) report 2013', p. 2.

230.	The most commonly cited . . .: ABS, '4364.0.55.007 – Australian Health Survey: Nutrition First Results – Foods and Nutrients, 2011–2012', media release, 9 May 2014, p. 2.

230.	Donovan revealed that . . .: Megan Miller, 'Chefs turn to tailors to suit modern demands', Herald Sun, 27 February 2016, http://www.heraldsun.com.au/lifestyle/mfwf/melbourne-food-and-wine-festival-allergies-off-menu/news-story/239ea470690ae8737d437b24aff68d4f

230.	According to market research firm . . .: International Markets Bureau (Canada), 'Global pathfinder report: food intolerance products', Agriculture and Agri-Food Canada, Ottawa, September 2012, www5.agr.gc.ca/resources/prod/Internet-Internet/MISB-DGSIM/ATS-SEA/PDF/6256-eng.pdf

231.	More than 130 different diseases . . .: Yehuda Shoenfeld et al., 'The autoimmunologist: geoepidemiology, a new center of gravity, and prime time for autoimmunity', Journal of Autoimmunity, 2008, vol. 31, no. 4, pp. 325–30.

231.	Individually, these conditions . . .: ASCIA, 'Allergy and immune diseases in Australia (AIDA) report 2013', p. 2.

232.	Zonulin release is triggered . . .: Alessio Fasano, 'Zonulin and its regulation of intestinal barrier function: the biological door to inflammation, autoimmunity, and cancer', American Physiological Review, 2011, vol. 9, no. 1, pp. 151–75, physrev.physiology.org/content/91/1/151.long

232.	Given the possible role of intestinal . . .: Fasano, 'Surprises from celiac disease'.

233.	One 2015 study demonstrated . . .: David Zeevi et al., 'Personalized nutrition by prediction of glycemic responses', Cell, 2015, vol. 163, no. 5, pp. 1079–94, www.cell.com/cell/fulltext/S0092-8674(15)01481-6

236.	In her opening address . . .: Dr Margaret Chan, Director General of the World Health Organization, Opening address at the 8th Global Conference on Health Promotion, Helsinki, Finland, 10 June 2013, 'WHO Director-General addresses health promotion conference', WHO, www.who.int/dg/speeches/2013/health_promotion_20130610/en

237.	Furnival had been co-principal . . .: Richard Mulgan, 'Furnival affair exposes the advisers' "accountability black hole" as a myth', 4 March 2014, www.canberratimes.com.au/national/public-service/furnival-affair-exposes-the-advisers-accountability-black-hole-as-a-myth-20140301-33t5g.html

238.	According to media reports . . .: Amy Corderoy, 'Staffer Alastair Furnival had links to alcohol industry, helped strip funding from group minimising alcohol harm', Sydney Morning Herald, 17 February 2014, www.smh.com.au/federal-politics/political-news/staffer-alastair-furnival-had-links-to-alcohol-industry-helped-strip-funding-from-group-minimising-alcohol-harm-20140217-32w0q.html

238.	Templeman also noted . . .: Corderoy, 'Staffer Alastair Furnival had links to alcohol industry, helped strip funding from group minimising alcohol harm'.

238.	'Health advisor' Furnival . . .: Mark Kenny & Amy Corderoy, 'Alastair Furnival lobbied the Tasmanian government to secure taxpayer funds for chocolate maker

Cadbury', *Sydney Morning Herald*, 21 February 2014, www.smh.com.au/federal-politics/political-news/alastair-furnival-lobbied-the-tasmanian-government-to-secure-taxpayer-funds-for-chocolate-maker-cadbury-20140220-334by.html

238. In a move that could be attributed . . .: Ibid.

238. Once exposed, however, Furnival . . .: Susan McDonald, 'Assistant Health Minister Fiona Nash's chief of staff Alastair Furnival resigns after conflict of interest claims', ABC News, 25 February 2014, www.abc.net.au/news/2014–02–14/staffer-at-centre-of-food-labelling-controversy-resigns/5261052

239. Some sugary breakfast cereals . . .: Cosima Marriner, 'Food brands "game" governments' health star rating scheme', *Sydney Morning Herald*, 14 February 2016, www.smh.com.au/national/food-brands-game-governments-health-star-rating-scheme-20160212-gmsuq0.html

239. It also allowed Pizza Cutters . . .: Rosie Squires, 'The tick that broke heart of foundation', *Sunday Telegraph*, 25 September 2011, www.theaustralian.com.au/news/the-tick-that-broke-heart-of-foundation/story-e6frg6n6-1226145340644

239. While the Australian Heart Foundation . . .: Ibid.

239. After a 2014 social media campaign . . .: 'Petition from Jessie Reimers delivered to Heart Foundation', Heart Foundation, 14 October 2014, heartfoundation.org.au/news/petition-from-jessie-reimers-delivered-to-heart-foundation

239. By the end of . . .: 'Thank you Tick for the past 26 years . . .', Heart Foundation, 8 December 2015, www.heartfoundation.org.au/news/thank-you-tick

240. In one of a damning series of emails . . .: Associated Press, 'Excerpts from emails between Coke, anti-obesity group', 25 November 2015, at finance.yahoo.com/news/excerpts-emails-between-coke-anti-080635667.html

240. While in response to the leaks Coca-Cola trotted out . . .: Anahad O'Connor, 'Coca-Cola's top obesity scientist departs amid murky research claims', *The Age*, 25 November 2015, www.smh.com.au/business/cocacolas-top-obesity-scientist-departs-amid-murky-research-claims-20151125-gl7gvl.html

241. For example, healthcare professionals . . .: Weaver et al., 'Processed foods: contributions to nutrition'.

241. Examples listed in order included . . .: 'Low Protein Diets and Renal Disease', Renal Resource Centre, Darling Point NSW, 2001.

242. As Margaret Chan points out . . .: Chan, Opening address at the 8th Global Conference on Health Promotion.

9 The rise and rise of the wellness industry

245. The term 'antifragile' was coined . . .: Nassim Nicholas Taleb, *Antifragile: Things That Gain From Disorder*, Penguin, London, 2012.

245. The 'antifragile' is curious . . .: Ibid., pp. 23–26

245. 'Antifragility is *beyond* resilience . . .: Ibid., p. 3.

246. For example: The medical fragilista . . .: Ibid., pp. 10–11.

247. Further supporting this idea . . .: Martin Raymond, *The Trendforecaster's Handbook*, Laurence King, London, 2010, p. 208.

248. According to research by the agency . . .: SRI International, 'The global spa and wellness Economy', Global Spa & Wellness Summit, Miami, September 2014, www.globalwellnesssummit.com/images/stories/gsws2014/presentations/Katherine-Johnston-Presentation.pdf

248. This industry cluster comprises four sectors . . .: Global Wellness Institute, 'Global Spa & Wellness Economy Monitor', Global Spa & Wellness Summit, Miami, September 2014, http://www.globalwellnesssummit.com/images/stories/gsws2014/pdf/GWI_Global_Spa_and_Wellness_Economy_Monitor_Full_Report_Final.pdf

248. The growth of the global . . .: 'Projected revenue growth rates of the global pharmaceutical industry from 2015 to 2018, by region', Statista, www.statista.com/statistics/398223/prediction-of-pharmaceutical-industry-cagr-worldwide-by-region

248. A comprehensive report . . .: Soeren Mattke et al., 'Workplace wellness programs study: final report', RAND Corporation, Santa Monica, California, 2013, www.rand.org/content/dam/rand/pubs/research_reports/RR200/RR254/RAND_RR254.pdf

249. According to a survey . . .: IFTF, 'The future of health and wellness in food retailing: forecasts and implications', IFTF, Palo Alto, California, April 2008, p. 6, www.iftf.org/our-work/health-self/health-horizons/the-future-of-health-and-wellness-in-food-retailing

250. In 2007, the Institute for the Future . . .: 'The Biocitizen and New Media Technologies Conference', Institute for the Future, May 2007, http://www.iftf.org/uploads/media/BiocitizensFINAL.pdf

252. According to the global internet rankings . . .: 'Top 500 sites on the web', Alexa, 12 August 2015, www.alexa.com/topsites/category/Top/Health/Nutrition

254. In 2015, it held its sixth . . .: Quantified Self, 'Quantified Self Expo 2015 Program', 20 June 2015, Fort Mason Centre, San Francisco, qs15.quantifiedself.com/expoprogram.pdf

255. Many biocitizens are interested . . .: 'The Biocitizen and New Media Technologies Conference', Institute for the Future.

257. At the time of writing, consumer genomics . . .: Ibid.

258. McCauley's data also . . .: Bamini Gopinath et al., 'Homocysteine, folate, vitamin B-12, and 10-y incidence of age related macular degeneration', *American Journal of Clinical Nutrition*, 2013, vol. 98, no. 1, pp. 129–35, ajcn.nutrition.org/content/98/1/129.full

259. He now takes L-methylfolate . . .: Elie Dolgin, 'Personalised investigation', *Nature Medicine*, 2010, vol. 16, no. 9, www.nature.com/nm/journal/v16/n9/full/nm0910-953.html

260. According to global research . . .: 'We are what we eat: healthy eating trends around the world', January 2015, Nielsen, New York, https://www.nielsen.com/content/dam/nielsenglobal/eu/nielseninsights/pdfs/Nielsen%20Global%20Health%20and%20Wellness%20Report%20-%20January%202015.pdf

261. Australia has GMO-labelling laws . . .: 'GM food labelling', Food Standards, August 2013, http://www.foodstandards.gov.au/consumer/gmfood/labelling/pages/default.aspx

261. Retail sales for organic products . . .: 'The world's largest market for organic products: organic retail sales value by country in 2013', Statista, 30 July 2015, www.statista.com/chart/3681/organic-retail-sales-value-by-country

263. Agricultural chemical company . . .: Niamh Michail, 'Bread companies should drop glyphosate, says Soil Association', Food Navigator, 20 July 2015, www.foodnavigator.com/Policy/Bread-companies-should-drop-glyphosate-says-Soil-Association

264. Commenting on the 2015 closures . . .: Candice Choi, 'APNewsBreak: McDonalds to shrink in US, 1st time in decades', Associated Press, 18 June 2015, bigstory.ap.org/article/fba7276a0e4241fda7dac7cacd505722/apnewsbreak-mcdonalds-shrinks-us-perhaps-1st-time

265. Paul Surman, president . . .: Serena Ng & Jonathan D. Rockoff, 'With top lines drooping, firms reach for vitamins', *Wall Street Journal*, 31 March 2013, www.wsj.com/articles/SB10001424127887324392804578362073624344816

265. Reckitt Benckiser has also . . .: Christopher Weaver & Tess Stynes, 'Reckitt Benckiser buys Schiff Nutrition in $1.4 billion deal', *Wall Street Journal*, 21 November 2012, www.wsj.com/articles/SB10001424127887324851704578133561127121192

265. The share price of well-known . . .: Mark Hawthorne, 'Vitamin maker's healthy glow after $1.67b buyout', *The Age*, 18 September 2015.

266. Greg Behar, chief executive . . .: Michael J. de la Merced, 'Nestlé Health Science to invest $65 million in a biotech start-up', *New York Times*, 6 January 2015, dealbook.nytimes.com/2015/01/06/nestle-health-sciences-to-invest-65-million-in-a-boston-biotech-start-up

266. Rather than relying . . .: Susie Ellis & Renee Moorefield, '2015: the year of the Ministry of Wellness?' Huffington Post, 13 January 2015, www.huffingtonpost.com/susie-ellis/2015-the-year-of-the-ministry-of-wellness_b_6438622.html

266. 'We will do whatever it takes . . .': Helen Andrews, 'India's prime minister wants the world to make ayurveda a way of life', Spa Opportunities, 24 November 2014, www.spaopportunities.com/detail.cfm?pagetype=detail&subject=news&codeID=312758

10 Mother Nature obeyed

272. To ensure only sustainable sources . . .: Paul Craig, 'Sustainable Seafood Guide', Australian Marine Conservation Society Inc, iTunes, 13 October 2015, https://itunes.apple.com/au/app/sustainable-seafood-guide/id461656264?mt=8

279. Today, many women would be . . .: Sevilay Temel et al., 'Knowledge of preconceptional folic acid supplementation and intention to seek for preconception care among men and women in an urban city: a population-based cross sectional study', *BMB Pregnancy and Childbirth*, 2015, https://www.ncbi.nlm.nih.gov/pmc/articles/PMC4684618/

279. Obesity from poor diet affects . . .: April L. Dawson et al., 'Maternal exposures in the National Birth Defects Prevention Study: time trends of selected exposures', *Birth Defects Res A Clin Mol Teratol*, August 2015, vol. 103, no. 8, pp. 703–712.

280. Statistics from the United Kingdom . . .: Linda Bryder, 'Breastfeeding and health professionals in Britain, New Zealand and the United States, 1900–1970', *Medical History*, 2005, vol. 49, no. 2, pp. 179–96, www.ncbi.nlm.nih.gov/pmc/articles/PMC1088218

281. The World Health Organization now . . .: WHO, 'Report of a WHO technical consultation on birth spacing', WHO Geneva, 13–15 June 2005, p. 2, www.who.int/maternal_child_adolescent/documents/birth_spacing.pdf?ua=1

282. In Australia, the experts tell us . . .: Brigid O'Connell, B., 'Sun protection top priority, even for those with vitamin D deficiency, warn experts', *Herald Sun*, 31 January 2016, p. 26, www.heraldsun.com.au/news/victoria/sun-protection-top-priority-even-for-those-with-vitamin-d-deficiency-warn-experts/news-story/82b9be3 3141f585e603356d5073df9f7

Index

highly unsaturated fatty acids 127–128, 134–136
HIIT (high-intensity interval training) 118–119
Hill, Professor James O. 240
Hippocratic Oath 81
HIV/AIDS 69–70
HLA-DQ genes 107
homocysteine 258
Honduras 171
hospitals *see* doctors and hospitals
HTT (huntingtin gene) 91–92
HUFAs (highly unsaturated fatty acids) 127–128, 134–136
human brain
    in adolescents 144
    gluten and 183–185
human disease types 90–91
human genome information 256
Human Genome Project 85, 88–90
human genome wellness testing 112–120
human life, seven requirements for 88
human microbiome 84, 102–104, 288
    adult microbiome 107–110
    consumers' viewpoint 235–236
    diversity and health 110–112
    fermented whole foods 276–277
    of indigenous peoples 108–110
    infant health and 104–107
Human Microbiome Project 102–104, 109
human physiology 1, 2
humans as diploid species 89
hunter-gatherers 1, 2, 109, 191
Huntington disease 91–92
hydrogenation 130
hypercalcaemia 193
hyperglycaemia 199

I
I Quit Sugar (Wilson) 219, 228
IgA nephropathy 7–8
immune system 103–104, 145–146, 158–159
In Defence of Food (Pollan) 216
India
    AYUSH Minister 266
    diabetes rates 34–35, 187–188
    Monsanto in 263
Indiana University 201
indigenous Australians *see also* Torres Strait Islanders
    cancer rates 167–168

chronic disease rates 26
reversibility of bad diet effects 24, 224
skin cancer 282
traditional foods 23, 24
tuberculosis death rates 13, 18–23, 158
type 2 diabetes rates 14
Weston Price's findings 18–19
indigenous peoples
    absence of cancer 31–32
    Australians *see* indigenous Australians
    bone problems 146
    distress at loss of health 16–17, 227
    effects of store staples on 12–13, 121–122, 176
    enforced labour of 152
    exposome 95–96, 110
    gluten and schizophrenia 184
    immunity in isolated *vs.* modernised 12–13
    increased susceptibility to pathogens 158
    microbiome 108–110
    pregnant women 279
    reversibility of bad diet effects 24, 224
    traditional foods 21–24
infectious diseases 188
infertility 162
    among African women slaves 153
    endocannabinoid system and 141–142
inflammation 162, 164–166
inflammatory bowel disease 182, 187
influenza 93, 159
information age 244
information race 215
information war 215, 235
Ingenio San Antonio 171–173
Ingham's 239
InsideTracker 255
Institute for the Future (Palo Alto) 225–226, 249–250
insulin resistance 33, 35, 203
insulin-like growth factor (IFG-1) 35
Intensive Dietary Management Program 203
International Federation of Clinical Chemistry Committee on Analytical Quality 224
the internet digital archive 15–16

The Shareholder Value Myth (Stout)
68–69
Sheffield Institute of Gluten-Related
Disorders 183
Shkreli, Martin 69–70
Shoenfeld, Professor Yehuda 75, 253
Shrapnel, Bill 218–219
Siberia 139
sickle cell anaemia 91
sickness industry 61–81
SIDS (sudden infant death syndrome)
107
Sikaris, Dr Ken 224
silica in foods 41
silicon dioxide 41
Sinclair, Upton 238
skin cancer 282
skin microbiota 110
slavery
abolitionists 153–154
sugar-cane workers 170–173
Trans-Atlantic slave trade 151–154
sleep problems 259–260
sleep trackers 255
slow food movement 261–262
SNPedia 257
SNPs (single-nucleotide
polymorphisms) 94–95, 114–115,
116, 257–259
soap operas 130
social change 51–52
social media 215–218
social networking 250–254
socioeconomic class 43
soft commodities 44
soft drinks see sugar drinks
soil depletion 117
soil quality 274–275
Sokolof, Phil 132–133
Solomon Islands 184
South Sea Islanders see Pacific Islanders
soy lecithin 170
soybeans
agglutinins from 189
as bulk commodity 44
genetically engineered 42
soybean products 42
soybean oil 122
blending hydrogenated cottonseed
oil with 123, 127, 130
consumption rates 125–126
linoleic acid in 122, 124–125,
186–187

market 33
omega-3 and omega-6 content 127
omega-3 and omega-6 ratio 125–126
soybean/cottonseed (trans fat) 123,
127, 130
spa industry 248
sprouted seeds 273
SRI International 248
Standard Oil 63
Stanton, Rosemary 222
Staphylococcus aureus 93, 107, 159
starch as carbohydrates 198
Stephen, Louise [author]
career 5–8, 66–67
as dialysis patient 241–242
diet 10
genome wellness testing 112–120
health 6
iron levels 192–193
kidney damage 7–9
kidney transplant 9–10
pregnancy 7–8
Stout, Lynn 68–69, 70, 79, 80
Strategic Issues Management 238
strategic philanthropy 63
stress response 115
Strine Jnr, Hon. Leo E. 70–71, 80
stroke 29
Stroke Foundation, Australia 207
sucrose 154–155, 163, 198
Sudler & Hennessey 207
sugars 151–173, 289
in breastmilk 106
cancer and 167–168
as carbohydrates 197–198
in combination with wheat
208–210
consumption rates 57
description 154–155, 163
effects on indigenous peoples 12–13,
121–122
genome wellness testing 114–115
gut bacteria and 108
intestinal permeability 170
John Yudkin and sugar problem
155–158, 211, 291
metabolic syndrome and 161–164
peripheral nerve damage and
164–166
sustainability and 206
telomere damage 166–167
tooth decay 159–161
zinc absorption and 117

MORE BESTSELLING NON-FICTION FROM PAN MACMILLAN

David Gillespie
The Eat Real Food Cookbook

'My wife, Lizzie, and our six kids have been living off the recipes and tips you're about to read for the better part of the last decade. This is an intensely practical book designed to solve an intensely practical problem: how to create high-quality food free of the twin evils of sugar and seed oils.'

For nearly ten years, David Gillespie has warned us of the dangers of sugar, and Australia has listened. More recently he has alerted us to the other toxin in our food supply: seed oil. Most processed food – from French fries to yoghurt to spreadable butter – contains one or both of these ingredients, so the question is: how do we eat real food?

Expanding on his 2015 bestseller *Eat Real Food*, David shows us how to:
- Identify and avoid sugar- and seed-oil-laden supermarket products
- Identify and shop for the healthy options
- Make the foods we normally buy in jars and packets – from mayonnaise to bread to tomato sauce
- Make simple, inexpensive daily meals the entire family will love
- Pack and plan for meals away from home
- Create healthier treats for all occasions, from kids' birthdays to cocktail parties

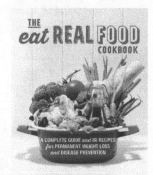

The Eat Real Food Cookbook is your guide to saying 'no' to the food that manufacturers want you to eat and 'yes' to the sort of food that will help you manage your weight and the long-term health of your family.

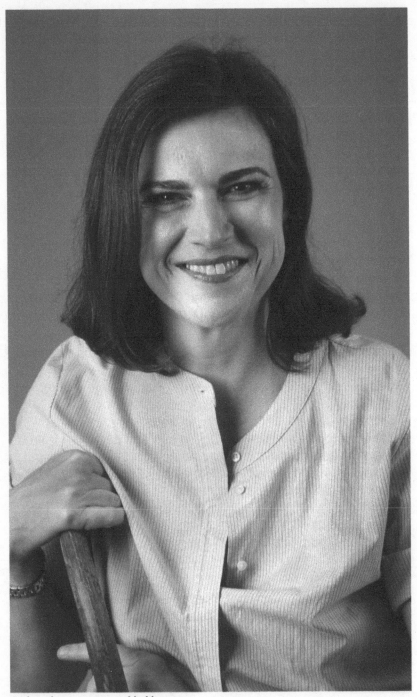
Author photo: cameronanddodd.com.au